SURGERY SOURCEBOOK

SIXTH EDITION

Health Reference Series

SURGERY SOURCEBOOK

SIXTH EDITION

Basic Consumer Health Information about Surgery, Its Types, and Future Trends, Common Surgeries and Procedures, such as Brain and Spinal Cord Tumor Surgery, Cataract Surgery, Breast Biopsy, Joint Replacement Surgery, Appendectomy, Uterine Fibroid Surgery, Circumcision, and Amputation Surgeries

Along with Information on Plastic and Reconstructive Surgery, Tips on Preparing for Surgery, Managing Postoperative Pain and Surgical Complications, Recovery and Rehabilitation after Surgery, a Glossary of Related Terms, and a Directory of Resources for Additional Help and Information

OMNIGRAPHICS
An imprint of Infobase

* * *

OMNIGRAPHICS
An imprint of Infobase
8 The Green
Suite #19225
Dover, DE 19901
www.infobase.com
James Chambers, *Editorial Director*

* * *

ISBN 978-0-7808-2142-2
E-ISBN 978-0-7808-2143-9

Library of Congress Cataloging-in-Publication Data

Names: Chambers, James (Editor), editor.

Title: Surgery sourcebook / edited by James Chambers.

Description: Sixth edition. | Dover, DE: Omnigraphics, an imprint of Infobase, [2024] | Series: Health reference series | Includes index. | Summary: "Provides basic consumer health information about common surgical procedures, tips on preparing for surgery, potential risks and complications, pain control options, along with facts about recovery and rehabilitation after surgery. Includes an index, glossary of related terms, and other resources"-- Provided by publisher.

Identifiers: LCCN 2024017118 (print) | LCCN 2024017119 (ebook) | ISBN 9780780821422 | ISBN 9780780821439 (eISBN)

Subjects: LCSH: Surgery--Popular works. | Consumer education--Popular works.

Classification: LCC RD31.3 .S87 2024 (print) | LCC RD31.3 (ebook) | DDC 617--dc23/eng/20240524

LC record available at https://lccn.loc.gov/2024017118

LC ebook record available at https://lccn.loc.gov/2024017119

Printed in the United States

Table of Contents

Part 3. Common Surgeries and Procedures

Part 4. Managing Postoperative Pain and Complications

Preface

ABOUT THIS BOOK

People undergo surgery for many reasons, including pain relief, disease treatment, and improved bodily function. In many cases, surgery can be life-saving, but it also carries risks such as bleeding, anesthesia side effects, and infection. Advances in surgical techniques, including lasers, robotic systems, and laparoscopic procedures, have helped reduce complications and enhance patient outcomes.

Surgery Sourcebook, Sixth Edition provides comprehensive information on various types of surgeries, including those involving the head and neck, eyes, dental and oral structures, breasts, cardiovascular system, joints and spine, gastrointestinal tract, and urological systems. It also covers weight-loss (bariatric), gynecologic, obstetric, and organ transplantation surgeries. The book offers guidance on preparing for surgery, such as choosing the right hospital, getting a second opinion, and understanding prehabilitation. It also addresses pain management, infection prevention, and strategies for recovery and rehabilitation post-surgery. The book concludes with a glossary of related terms and a directory of resources for additional help and information.

HOW TO USE THIS BOOK

This book is divided into parts and chapters. Parts focus on broad areas of interest. Chapters are devoted to single topics within a part.

Part 1: Introduction to Surgery provides foundational information about various types of surgeries, including specialized techniques such as laparoscopy, robotically-assisted systems, laser, and cryosurgery. This part concludes with insights into future trends in surgical practices.

Part 2: Preparing for Surgery offers essential guidance for patients on selecting a hospital, obtaining a second opinion, and understanding preoperative procedures. It also details the services provided by ambulatory surgical centers and includes information on advance care planning and patient safety.

Part 3: Common Surgeries and Procedures covers a wide range of surgical procedures, including those related to the head and neck, eyes, dental and oral structures, breasts, cardiovascular system, joints and spine, gastrointestinal tract, urological systems, and more. This part also discusses weight-loss (bariatric), gynecologic, obstetric, plastic, and reconstructive surgeries, along with organ transplantation and amputation procedures.

Part 4: Managing Postoperative Pain and Complications focuses on addressing and preventing postoperative complications. It covers pain management, blood loss control, and the prevention of health-care-associated infections (HAIs) such as surgical site infections (SSIs), catheter-associated urinary tract infections (CAUTIs), and methicillin-resistant *Staphylococcus aureus* (MRSA) infections. The part also discusses other potential complications, including abdominal adhesions, venous thromboembolism (VTE), and cardiogenic shock.

Part 5: Recovery and Rehabilitation after Surgery provides insights into the recovery process following surgery, including the use of ventilation support and strategies for caring for incisions, surgical drains, and blood clot risks. Detailed information on hospital discharge planning and transitioning to post-surgical care is also provided.

Part 6: Additional Help and Information includes a glossary of important terms related to surgery and a directory of organizations that offer information and support for people undergoing surgery and their caregivers.

BIBLIOGRAPHIC NOTE

This volume contains documents and excerpts from publications issued by the following U.S. government agencies: Agency for Healthcare Research and Quality (AHRQ); Centers for Disease Control and Prevention (CDC); Centers for Medicare & Medicaid Services (CMS); Effective Health Care Program; *Eunice Kennedy Shriver* National Institute of Child Health and Human Development (NICHD); Health Resources and Services Administration (HRSA); MedlinePlus; National Aeronautics and Space Administration (NASA); National Cancer Institute (NCI); National Eye Institute (NEI); National Heart, Lung, and Blood Institute (NHLBI); National Institute of Arthritis and Musculoskeletal and Skin Diseases (NIAMS); National Institute of Biomedical Imaging and Bioengineering (NIBIB); National Institute of Dental and Craniofacial Research (NIDCR); National Institute of Diabetes and Digestive and Kidney Diseases (NIDDK); National Institute of Neurological Disorders and Stroke (NINDS); National Institute on Aging

(NIA); National Institute on Deafness and Other Communication Disorders (NIDCD); *NIH News in Health*; Office of Disease Prevention and Health Promotion (ODPHP); Office on Women's Health (OWH); Surveillance, Epidemiology, and End Results (SEER) Program; U.S. Department of Veterans Affairs (VA); and U.S. Food and Drug Administration (FDA).

ABOUT THE *HEALTH REFERENCE SERIES*

The *Health Reference Series* is designed to provide basic medical information for patients, families, caregivers, and the general public. Each volume provides comprehensive coverage on a particular topic. This is especially important for people who may be dealing with a newly diagnosed disease or a chronic disorder in themselves or in a family member. People looking for preventive guidance, information about disease warning signs, medical statistics, and risk factors for health problems will also find answers to their questions in the *Health Reference Series*. The *Series*, however, is not intended to serve as a tool for diagnosing illness, in prescribing treatments, or as a substitute for the physician-patient relationship. All people concerned about medical symptoms or the possibility of disease are encouraged to seek professional care from an appropriate health-care provider.

A NOTE ABOUT SPELLING AND STYLE

Health Reference Series editors use *Stedman's Medical Dictionary* as an authority for questions related to the spelling of medical terms and *The Chicago Manual of Style* for questions related to grammatical structures, punctuation, and other editorial concerns. Consistent adherence is not always possible, however, because the individual volumes within the *Series* include many documents from a wide variety of different producers, and the editor's primary goal is to present material from each source as accurately as is possible. This sometimes means that information in different chapters or sections may follow other guidelines and alternate spelling authorities. For example, occasionally a copyright holder may require that eponymous terms be shown in possessive forms (Crohn's disease vs. Crohn disease) or that British spelling norms be retained (leukaemia vs. leukemia).

HEALTH REFERENCE SERIES UPDATE POLICY

The inaugural book in the *Health Reference Series* was the first edition of *Cancer Sourcebook* published in 1989. Since then, the *Series* has been enthusiastically received by librarians and in the medical community. In order to maintain the standard of providing high-quality health information for the layperson, the editorial staff felt it was necessary to implement a policy of updating volumes when warranted.

Medical researchers have been making tremendous strides, and it is the purpose of the *Health Reference Series* to stay current with the most recent advances. Each decision to update a volume is made on an individual basis. Some of the considerations include how much new information is available and the feedback we receive from people who use the books. If there is a topic you would like to see added to the update list, or an area of medical concern you feel has not been adequately addressed, please write to: custserv@infobaselearning.com.

Part 1 | Introduction to Surgery

Chapter 1 | Types of Surgery

Surgical procedures are essential to modern medicine, addressing various health conditions from diagnosis to treatment. These procedures not only assist in detecting diseases but also play a crucial role in their management and prevention. Advancements in surgical methods, from minimally invasive techniques to complex open surgeries, have greatly improved patient outcomes and recovery times. Understanding the various types of surgical procedures and their implications is essential for both patients and health-care providers in navigating the complexities of medical treatment.

DIAGNOSTIC SURGERY

There are many ways to detect or confirm the presence of cancer. Microscopic examination of biopsy samples is the ideal method for making a positive diagnosis. This procedure involves physically removing all or part of a suspected tumor (tissue, cells, or fluid) and examining this material under a microscope. The purpose of a biopsy is to identify the histologic type of cancer and possibly define the extent of the disease.

Any organ in the body can be biopsied using a variety of techniques. Some may require major surgery, while others may not even require local anesthesia. Types of biopsies include:

- bone marrow biopsy
- colposcopic biopsy
- core biopsy
- excisional biopsy
- endoscopic biopsy
- fine needle aspiration biopsy

- incisional biopsy
- stereotactic biopsy

With the exception of excisional biopsy, biopsies typically leave gross tumors in the body.

The diagram that follows differentiates between an incisional biopsy and an excisional biopsy. An incisional biopsy removes a small portion of the tumor to be analyzed by the pathologist to diagnose the cancer. An incisional biopsy is considered a surgical diagnostic and staging procedure. The results of the biopsy, if cancer is identified, diagnose the malignancy and, depending on specifics about the specimen, can contribute staging information.

An excisional biopsy of the primary site removes the entire tumor, plus a margin around the tumor. This procedure is considered a surgical procedure and treatment for the cancer. Often, the excisional biopsy may be the only surgical treatment the patient receives, as the entire tumor is resected in this procedure.

Different types of endoscopes may be used in performing diagnostic and surgical procedures. These include:

- arthroscope
- bronchoscope
- colonoscope
- colposcope
- cystoscope
- esophagoscope
- gastroscope
- laparoscope
- laryngoscope
- neuroendoscope
- proctoscope
- sigmoidoscope

These scopes may be used for both surgical and diagnostic procedures.[1]

---

[1] Surveillance, Epidemiology, and End Results (SEER) Program, "Diagnostic Surgery," National Cancer Institute (NCI), December 21, 2023. Available online. URL: https://training.seer.cancer.gov/treatment/surgery/types/diagnostic.html. Accessed June 19, 2024.

CURATIVE SURGERY

Curative surgery aims to remove all malignant (cancerous) tissue with the goal of curing the disease. This involves removing part or all of the cancerous organ or tissue, along with a small amount of healthy tissue around it. Nearby lymph nodes may also be removed during curative surgery. It is most effective for localized cancer. Sometimes, chemotherapy or radiation therapy is given before surgery to shrink the tumor or after surgery to eliminate any remaining cancer cells.[2]

PALLIATIVE SURGERY

In addition to diagnostic, primary, and preventive surgeries, surgical procedures are also performed to improve the patient's quality of life (QOL). Palliative surgery can restore function, reduce cancer burden, reduce pain by alleviating an obstruction, and reduce symptoms.

Cancer causes pain to most cancer patients, as does the treatment. It is estimated that 80 percent of cancer patients have two or more episodes of pain. More patients experience pain with advanced disease. The QOL for those in great pain, resulting from either the disease or the treatment, is greatly compromised. Under such circumstances, palliative surgery may be performed. For example, the procedure may involve the removal of a painful primary or metastatic tumor mass, such as a solitary spinal metastasis.

The purpose of palliative surgery is mainly to reduce pain and/or other symptoms (e.g., debulking to relieve bowel compression in a patient with ovarian cancer). The surgery may not eradicate cancer tissue in the patient. In fact, palliative surgery is often deemed worthwhile and feasible by cancer specialists when the disease is not responsive to any type of curative treatment. A successful palliative surgery may make the patient's life more comfortable and prolong their life. Palliative surgery that removes cancer tissue is recorded as cancer-directed surgery. Palliative surgery, such as a

[2] "Curative Surgery," National Cancer Institute (NCI), September 15, 2016. Available online. URL: www.cancer.gov/publications/dictionaries/cancer-terms/def/curative-surgery. Accessed June 19, 2024.

nerve block procedure to interrupt pain signals in the nervous system or a stent placement to alleviate obstruction, which does not remove cancer tissue, is not recorded as cancer-directed surgery.

A cancer registrar should record palliative procedures as non-cancer-directed surgery in the cancer abstract.[3]

PREVENTIVE SURGERY

In preventive surgery, the surgeon removes tissue that does not yet contain cancer cells but is likely to become cancerous in the future. This may also be referred to as "prophylactic surgery."

- **Example 1**. Based on genetic tests, a woman whose mother has ovarian cancer has a higher than average risk of developing ovarian cancer. After a thorough discussion and consideration with her physician, the woman elects to remove her ovaries to avoid the risk of ovarian cancer. The procedure is called "prophylactic oophorectomy" (removal of both ovaries).
- **Example 2**. A woman is diagnosed with breast cancer. Her history and physical examination indicate she has a strong family history of breast cancer. Her BRCA-1 genetic test returns positive. Her physician may decide to discuss a prophylactic mastectomy surgery with her to remove the opposite breast. The prophylactic mastectomy is intended to prevent a later cancer diagnosis in the opposite breast.
- **Example 3**. Patients who have a congenital or genetic trait that creates a high risk of developing cancer may benefit from preventive surgery. Studies have shown that half of the patients with familial polyposis of the colon, without a preventive colectomy, would develop cancer of the colon by age 40, and all would develop the disease by age 70.[4]

---

[3] Surveillance, Epidemiology, and End Results (SEER) Program, "Palliative Surgery," National Cancer Institute (NCI), December 21, 2023. Available online. URL: https://training.seer.cancer.gov/treatment/surgery/types/palliative.html. Accessed June 19, 2024.

[4] Surveillance, Epidemiology, and End Results (SEER) Program, "Preventive Surgery," National Cancer Institute (NCI), December 21, 2023. Available online. URL: https://training.seer.cancer.gov/treatment/surgery/types/palliative.html. Accessed June 19, 2024.

OPEN-HEART SURGERY

Heart surgeries are done in hospitals. Typically, they are performed by highly trained doctors called "cardiothoracic surgeons." A team of health-care providers, including your surgeon, imaging specialists, anesthesiologists, and nurses, will care for you during your hospital stay.

Depending on various factors, including your heart condition and overall health, your surgeon may perform minimally invasive heart surgery, off-pump surgery, or open-heart surgery. For example, coronary artery bypass graft surgery (CABG) can be performed using any of these methods. Your provider will work with you to decide which method is best based on how serious your heart problem is and any factors that may put you at risk for complications.

Open-heart surgery is any kind of surgery in which a surgeon makes a large incision in the chest to open the rib cage and operate on the heart. For this type of surgery, you will be given anesthesia to make you unconscious and unaware of pain.

Your surgeon will make a 6- to 8-inch incision down the center of your chest wall. They will then cut your breastbone and open your rib cage to reach your heart. You will receive medicine during the surgery to thin your blood and keep it from clotting. Your surgeon will connect a heart-lung bypass machine to your heart. The machine will take over your heart's pumping action and move blood away from your heart. This is done because surgeons can better perform some procedures on a heart that is not beating and does not have blood flowing through it.

Once the bypass machine starts to work, the surgeon will repair your heart problem. After the surgery is done, they will restore blood flow to your heart. Usually, your heart will start beating again on its own. Sometimes, mild electric shocks are used to restart the heart.[5]

MINIMALLY INVASIVE SURGERY

Surgery that is done using small incisions and a few stitches is called "minimally invasive surgery." During this type of surgery, one or more small incisions may be made in the body. A laparoscope, a

[5] "What to Expect during Surgery," National Heart, Lung, and Blood Institute (NHLBI), June 1, 2022. Available online. URL: www.nhlbi.nih.gov/health/heart-surgery/during. Accessed June 28, 2024.

thin tube-like instrument with a light and a lens for viewing, is inserted through one opening to guide the surgery. Tiny surgical instruments are inserted through other openings to perform the surgery. Minimally invasive surgery may cause less pain, scarring, and damage to healthy tissue, and the patient may have a faster recovery than with traditional surgery.[6]

ROBOTIC SURGERY

Different types of computer-assisted surgical systems can be used for pre-operative planning, surgical navigation, and assistance in performing surgical procedures. Robotically-assisted surgical (RAS) devices are one type of computer-assisted surgical system. Sometimes referred to as "robotic surgery," RAS devices enable the surgeon to use computer and software technology to control and move surgical instruments through one or more tiny incisions in the patient's body for various surgical procedures.

The benefits of an RAS device may include its ability to facilitate minimally invasive surgery and assist with complex tasks in confined areas of the body. The device is not actually a robot because it cannot perform surgery without direct human control.

RAS devices generally have several components, which may include:

- **Console**. Where the surgeon sits during surgery. The console is the control center of the device, allowing the surgeon to view the surgical field through a three-dimensional (3D) endoscope and control the movement of the surgical instruments.
- **Bedside cart**. Includes three or four hinged mechanical arms, a camera (endoscope), and surgical instruments that the surgeon controls during surgical procedures.
- **Separate cart**. Contains supporting hardware and software components, such as an electrosurgical unit (ESU), suction/irrigation pumps, and a light source for the endoscope.

[6] "Minimally Invasive Surgery," National Cancer Institute (NCI), September 13, 2016. Available online. URL: www.cancer.gov/publications/dictionaries/cancer-terms/def/minimally-invasive-surgery. Accessed June 28, 2024.

Most surgeons use multiple surgical instruments and accessories with the RAS device, such as scalpels, forceps, graspers, dissectors, cautery, scissors, retractors, and suction irrigators.

Common Uses of Robotically-Assisted Surgical Devices

The U.S. Food and Drug Administration (FDA) has cleared RAS devices for use by trained physicians in an operating room environment for laparoscopic surgical procedures in general surgery, cardiac, colorectal, gynecologic, head and neck, thoracic, and urologic surgical procedures. Some common procedures that may involve RAS devices are gallbladder removal, hysterectomy, and prostatectomy (removal of the prostate).

While robotically-assisted surgery is safe and effective for performing certain procedures when used appropriately and with proper training, the FDA has not granted marketing authorization for any RAS device system for use in the United States specifically for the prevention or treatment of cancer.[7]

GASTROINTESTINAL SURGERY

Severe obesity is a chronic condition that is difficult to treat through diet and exercise alone. Gastrointestinal surgery is an option for people who are severely obese and cannot lose weight by traditional means or who suffer from serious obesity-related health problems. The operation promotes weight loss by restricting food intake and, in some cases, interrupting the digestive process. As with other treatments for obesity, the best results are achieved with healthy eating behaviors and regular physical activity.

Gastrointestinal surgery for obesity, also called "bariatric surgery," alters the digestive process. The operations can be divided into three types: restrictive, malabsorptive, and combined restrictive/malabsorptive. Restrictive operations limit food intake by creating a narrow passage from the upper part of the stomach into the larger lower part, reducing the amount of food the stomach

[7] "Computer-Assisted Surgical Systems," U.S. Food and Drug Administration (FDA), June 21, 2022. Available online. URL: www.fda.gov/medical-devices/surgery-devices/computer-assisted-surgical-systems. Accessed June 28, 2024.

can hold and slowing the passage of food through the stomach. Malabsorptive operations do not limit food intake but instead exclude most of the small intestine from the digestive tract, so fewer calories and nutrients are absorbed. Malabsorptive operations, also called "intestinal bypasses," are no longer recommended because they result in severe nutritional deficiencies. Combined operations use stomach restriction and a partial bypass of the small intestine.[8]

NEUROSURGERY

Surgery is usually the first treatment to both obtain tissue for diagnosis and remove as much tumor as can be done safely. Surgery may be the only treatment you need if your tumor is considered benign or low-grade. Based on the type and grade (low versus high), doctors often recommend follow-up treatment, including radiation and chemotherapy, or an experimental treatment. You will be referred to specialists to provide guidance on this treatment.

Surgery is usually the first step in treating an accessible tumor—one that can be removed without risking neurological damage. Many low-grade tumors and secondary (metastatic) cancerous tumors can be removed entirely. Some tumors have a clearly defined shape and can be removed more easily. Your surgeon will try removing (resecting or excising) all or as much of the tumor as possible. For malignant central nervous system (CNS) tumors, this is best performed by a neurosurgeon.

An inaccessible or inoperable tumor is one that cannot be removed surgically because of the risk of severe nervous system damage during the operation. These tumors are frequently located deep within the brain or near vital structures such as the brain stem and may not have well-defined edges. In these cases, a biopsy may be performed.

A biopsy is sometimes performed to diagnose and help doctors determine how to treat a tumor. A biopsy is performed by inserting

[8] "Gastrointestinal Surgery for Severe Obesity," National Institute of Diabetes and Digestive and Kidney Diseases (NIDDK), December 2004. Available online. URL: www.govinfo.gov/content/pkg/GOVPUB-HE20-PURL-LPS78258/pdf/GOVPUB-HE20-PURL-LPS78258.pdf. Accessed June 28, 2024.

a needle through a small hole in the body and taking a small piece of the tumor tissue. A pathologist examines the tissue for certain changes that signal cancer and determines its stage or grade.

In some cases, a surgeon may need to insert a shunt into the skull to drain any dangerous buildup of cerebrospinal fluid (CSF) caused by the tumor. A shunt is a flexible plastic tube that diverts the flow of CSF from the central nervous system to another part of the body, where it can be absorbed as part of the normal circulatory process.

During surgery, some tools used in the operating room include a surgical microscope, an endoscope (a small viewing tube attached to a video camera), and miniature precision instruments that allow surgery to be performed through a small incision in the brain or spine. Other tools include:

- **Intraoperative MRI**. This uses a special type of MRI to provide real-time monitoring and evaluation of the surgery. Constantly updated images let doctors see how much of the tumor has been removed.
- **Navigation equipment**. Used in computer-guided, or stereotactic, neurosurgery, this gives doctors a precise, 3D map of the spine or brain as the operation progresses. A computer uses pre-operative diagnostic images to reduce the risk of damage to surrounding tissue.
- **Intraoperative nerve monitoring tests**. These use real-time recordings of nerve cell activity to determine the role of specific nerves and to monitor brain activity as the surgery progresses.

Some surgeries may occur while the individual is awake under monitored anesthesia care, rather than under general anesthesia. This allows doctors to monitor the individual's speech and motor functions as a tumor is being removed.[9]

[9] "Brain and Spinal Cord Tumors," National Institute of Neurological Disorders and Stroke (NINDS), November 28, 2023. Available online. URL: www.ninds.nih.gov/health-information/disorders/brain-and-spinal-cord-tumors. Accessed June 28, 2024.

ORTHOPEDIC SURGERY

Types of Procedures and Services

- **Joint replacement**. Hip, knee, and shoulder replacements, including the innovative anterior hip approach and same-day joint replacement.
- **Tendon and ligament repairs**. Hand, elbow, shoulder, hip, and knee repairs (both basic and complex).
- **Fracture repair**. Treating broken bones.
- **Arthroscopic surgery**. Minimally invasive procedures for the shoulder, knee, elbow, and wrist.
- **Musculoskeletal tumor treatment**. It involves specialized procedures to remove tumors from bones and soft tissues, ensuring the preservation of limb function and overall health.
- **Total joint replacement**. This surgery is for patients with debilitating joint pain due to osteoarthritis in the shoulder, hip, or knee. Surgeons replace worn-out joint surfaces with alloy metal and durable plastic materials. People who have exhausted non-operative measures may opt for this procedure.

What to Expect

- Your surgical team includes orthopedic surgeons, nurses, technicians, and an anesthesiologist.
- During surgery, the arthritic joint surface is precisely removed, and new metal and plastic surfaces are implanted for pain-free motion.

Recovery

- You will receive personalized care instructions.
- Blood clot prevention measures (such as aspirin) are recommended.
- Visiting nurses and physical therapists provide home care during the initial weeks after surgery.[10]

[10] "Orthopedic Surgery at VA Boston Healthcare," U.S. Department of Veterans Affairs (VA), November 20, 2023. Available online. URL: www.va.gov/boston-health-care/programs/orthopedic-surgery-at-va-boston-healthcare. Accessed June 28, 2024.

PLASTIC AND RECONSTRUCTIVE SURGERY

- **Reconstructive surgery**. Performed on abnormal body structures caused by congenital defects, developmental abnormalities, trauma, infection, tumors, or disease. It is generally performed to improve function but may also be done to approximate a normal appearance.
- **Cosmetic surgery**. Performed to reshape normal structures of the body to improve the patient's appearance and self-esteem. Corrective facial surgery will be considered cosmetic rather than reconstructive when there is no functional impairment present. If a non-covered cosmetic surgery is performed in the same operative period as a covered surgical procedure, benefits will be provided for the covered surgical procedure only. Benefits may be provided for complications arising from cosmetic surgery, including infection, hemorrhage, or other serious documented medical complications.[11]

[11] "Plastic Surgery," Centers for Medicare & Medicaid Services (CMS), April 2, 2020. Available online. URL: www.cms.gov/medicare-coverage-database/view/lcd.aspx?LCDId=37020&ContrId=345. Accessed June 28, 2024.

Chapter 2 | Surgery in Older Adults

In some cases, surgery may be the best treatment for older adults with certain conditions. If so, your doctor will refer you to a surgeon. Knowing more about the operation will help you make an informed decision about how to proceed. It also will help you get ready for the surgery, which improves your recovery.

Ask the surgeon to explain what will be done during the operation and what reading material, videos, or websites you can review before the procedure. For older adults, understanding the specifics of the surgery, including any age-related risks, is particularly important.

Find out if you will have to stay overnight in the hospital or if the surgery can be done on an outpatient basis, and if you will need someone to drive you home. Minor surgeries that do not require an overnight stay can sometimes be done at ambulatory surgical centers.

QUESTIONS TO ASK YOUR SURGEON

- What is the success rate of the operation? How many of these operations have you done successfully?
- What problems can occur with this surgery? What kind of pain or discomfort can I expect?
- What kind of anesthesia will I have? Are there any risks associated with its use in older people?
- Will I have to stay in the hospital overnight? How long is recovery expected to take? What does it involve? When can I get back to my normal routine?

GETTING A SECOND OPINION

When patients are diagnosed with a serious illness or surgery is recommended, they often seek a second opinion. Hearing the views of two different doctors can help you decide what is best for you. Your insurance plan may require it. Doctors are accustomed to this practice, and most will not be insulted by your request for a second opinion. Your doctor may even be able to suggest other doctors who can review your case.

Always check with your insurance provider in advance to find out if a second opinion is covered under your policy, if there are restrictions on which doctors you can see, and if you need a referral form from your primary doctor.

ASK ABOUT DIFFERENT TREATMENT OPTIONS

You will benefit most from treatment when you know what is happening and are involved in making decisions. Ensure you understand your treatment and what it will or will not do. Have the doctor give you written directions, and feel free to ask questions. For example, What are the pros and cons of having surgery at this stage? Or do I have any other choices?

If your doctor suggests a treatment that makes you uncomfortable, ask if other treatments might work. If cost is a concern, ask the doctor if cheaper choices are available. The doctor can work with you to develop a treatment plan that meets your needs.

Things to Remember When Deciding on a Treatment

- **Discuss different treatment choices.** There are various ways to manage many health conditions, especially chronic conditions such as high blood pressure (HBP) and cholesterol. Ask what your options are.
- **Discuss the risks and benefits of treatment options.** Once you know your options, ask about the pros and cons of each one. Find out what side effects might occur, how long the treatment would continue, and how likely the treatment will work for you.

- **Consider how a treatment may affect your life**. When thinking about the pros and cons of a treatment, do not forget to consider its effect on your overall life. For instance, will one of the side effects interfere with a regular activity that means a lot to you? Is one treatment choice expensive and not covered by your insurance? Doctors need to know about these practical matters, so they can work with you to develop a treatment plan that meets your needs.

QUESTIONS TO ASK ABOUT TREATMENT OPTIONS

- Are there any risks associated with the treatment?
- How soon should treatment start? How long will it last?
- Are there other treatments available?
- How much will the treatment cost? Will my insurance cover it?

TALKING WITH MEDICAL SPECIALISTS

Your doctor may send you to a specialist for further evaluation, or you may request to see a specialist yourself. Your insurance plan may require a referral from your primary doctor. A visit to the specialist may be short. Often, the specialist has already seen your medical records or test results and is familiar with your case. If you are unclear about what the specialist tells you, ask questions.

For example, if the specialist says you have a medical condition that you are not familiar with, you may want to say something such as I do not know much about that condition. Could you explain what it is and how it might affect me? Or I have heard that it is a painful problem. What can be done to prevent or manage the pain?

You may also ask for written materials to read, or you can call your primary doctor to clarify anything you don't understand.

Ask the specialist to send information about any diagnosis or treatment to your primary doctor. This allows your primary doctor to keep track of your medical care. You also should let your primary doctor know at your next visit how well any treatments or medications the specialist recommended are working.

QUESTIONS TO ASK YOUR SPECIALIST

- What is the diagnosis?
- What treatment do you recommend? How soon do I need to begin the new treatment?
- Will you discuss my care with my primary doctor?

DISCUSS HOW PREVENTION CAN IMPROVE YOUR HEALTH

Doctors and other health professionals may suggest that you change your diet, activity level, or other aspects of your life to help you manage medical conditions. Research has shown that these changes, particularly increased exercise, positively affect overall health.

Until recently, preventing disease in older people received little attention. But things are changing. We now know that it is never too late to stop smoking, improve your diet, or start exercising. Regular checkups and seeing other health-care professionals, such as dentists and eye specialists, help promote good health. Even people who have chronic diseases, such as arthritis or diabetes, can prevent further disability and, in some cases, control the progress of the disease.

If a certain disease or health condition runs in your family, ask your doctor if there are steps you can take to help prevent it. If you have a chronic condition, ask how you can manage it and if there are things you can do to keep it from worsening. If you want to discuss health and disease prevention with your doctor, say so when you make your next appointment. This lets the doctor plan to spend more time with you.

It is just as important to talk with your doctor about lifestyle changes as it is about treatment. For example, I know that you have told me to eat more dairy products, but they really disagree with me. Is there something else I could eat instead? Maybe an exercise class would help, but I cannot get to the senior center. Is there something else you could suggest?

As with treatments, consider all the alternatives, weigh the pros and cons, and remember to consider your own point of view. Tell your doctor if you feel her or his suggestions would not work for you and explain why. Keep talking with your doctor to develop a plan that works.

Many doctors now recommend that older people try to make physical activity a part of everyday life. When you are making your list of things to talk about with your doctor, add exercise. Ask how exercise would benefit you, if there are any activities you should avoid, and whether your doctor can recommend any specific kinds of exercise.

QUESTIONS TO ASK YOUR DOCTOR ABOUT PREVENTION

- Is there any way to prevent a condition in my family before it affects me?
- Are there ways to keep my condition from getting worse?
- How will making a change in my habits help me?
- Are there any risks in making this change?
- Are there support groups or community services that might help me?[1]

[1] National Institute on Aging (NIA), "Discussing Health Decisions with Your Doctor," National Institutes of Health (NIH), February 3, 2020. Available online. URL: www.nia.nih.gov/health/medical-care-and-appointments/discussing-health-decisions-your-doctor. Accessed April 8, 2024.

Chapter 3 | Specialized Surgical Techniques

Chapter Contents

Section 3.1 | Laparoscopy

WHAT IS A LAPAROSCOPY?

A laparoscopy is a type of surgery that allows a surgeon to look inside your body without making a large incision. It is used to help diagnose and sometimes treat conditions in the abdomen or pelvis.

To perform a laparoscopy, a surgeon makes a small cut near your belly button, usually less than a half-inch long. The surgeon inserts a long, thin tube with a camera through the cut and into your body. This tube is called a "laparoscope." The camera sends images from inside your body to a video monitor, allowing the surgeon to see inside your body.

The surgeon may make one or two other small cuts in your abdomen to insert special surgical tools. Using these tools, the surgeon can remove samples of tissue to check for signs of disease, known as a "biopsy."

Sometimes, during a laparoscopy, the surgeon will use these tools to perform procedures to treat specific problems. For example, if a tumor is found during the procedure, the surgeon may remove it during the same surgery. Many common surgical treatments can be performed with laparoscopic surgery.

Laparoscopy is sometimes called "minimally invasive surgery" or "keyhole surgery" because it requires smaller cuts than traditional, open surgery. The use of smaller cuts has several benefits, including shorter hospital stays, less pain, faster recovery, and smaller scars.

WHAT IS IT USED FOR?

Laparoscopy is used to help diagnose the cause of symptoms in the abdomen or pelvis. It is usually performed if imaging tests, such as x-rays, ultrasounds, and magnetic resonance imaging (MRI) scans, have not provided enough information to confirm a diagnosis.

The test is often used to help diagnose:

- digestive diseases
- urinary disorders
- disorders in the female reproductive system, including the uterus, ovaries, and fallopian tubes

A surgeon uses laparoscopy to:

- examine organs and glands to look for:
  - abnormal growths, such as cysts and tumors (cancerous and noncancerous)
  - scar tissue and adhesions
  - bleeding
  - infections
- collect tissue samples to check for disease
- determine if a known cancer has spread in the body

WHY DO YOU NEED A LAPAROSCOPY?

There are many reasons why you may need a laparoscopy, including if:

- You have pain or other symptoms in your abdomen or pelvis, and imaging tests have not been able to find the cause.
- You have been in a serious accident or have been wounded and may have organ injuries.
- You have cancer, and your health-care provider needs to know if it has spread to other parts of your body.
- You have had abnormal liver tests, and your provider does not know why.

If you are female, you may need a laparoscopy to:

- determine the cause of problems getting pregnant
- diagnose symptoms involving your reproductive organs, including:
  - pelvic inflammatory disease (PID)
  - endometriosis
  - ectopic pregnancy
  - uterine fibroids
  - ovarian cysts

WHAT HAPPENS DURING A LAPAROSCOPY?

Laparoscopy is usually done in a hospital or an outpatient clinic. In general, it includes these steps:

- You will wear a hospital gown and lie on an operating table.

- Usually, you will receive general anesthesia, which is medicine that makes you sleep during the surgery. The medicine is injected into your bloodstream through an intravenous (IV) line inserted into a vein. You may also inhale gas from a mask to make you sleep.
- To perform the laparoscopy, the surgeon will:
  - make a small cut near your belly button;
  - put carbon dioxide gas into your abdomen to open up space between your organs, making it easier to see them;
  - insert the laparoscope and small camera into your abdomen; and
  - move the laparoscope to look at your organs and glands on a computer screen.
- If you need a biopsy or another procedure, the surgeon may need to make more small cuts to insert surgical tools.
- When the surgeon is done, the tools and most of the gas will be removed from your body, and the small incisions will be closed and bandaged.
- After surgery, you will be moved to a recovery room. In most cases, you can go home after a few hours, depending on the procedures done during the laparoscopy. Before you leave, you will receive information about what to expect over the next few days at home.

PREPARING FOR A LAPAROSCOPY

Your provider will let you know how to prepare. Be sure to follow all instructions. You will need to fast (not eat or drink) for a period of time before a laparoscopy. Ask your provider whether to take your usual medicines and/or supplements, but do not stop taking any medicine without consulting your provider first.

Plan to wear loose-fitting clothes because your abdomen may be bloated from the gas and a little sore after the surgery. You are also likely to feel groggy, so you must arrange for someone to take you home.

ARE THERE ANY RISKS TO THE TEST?

You may experience mild abdominal pain or discomfort for a few days after a laparoscopy. You may also have neck or shoulder pain, as the gas used in the surgery can irritate nerves in your abdomen that run through your shoulder.

Serious problems after a laparoscopy are uncommon, but they can include bleeding, infection, blood clots, damage to an organ or blood vessel, and complications from the anesthesia.

WHAT DO THE RESULTS MEAN?

The results of a laparoscopy depend on the reason for the procedure. Your provider can explain what was found and what that information means for your health. In general, your provider will be able to make a very accurate diagnosis of your condition based on the information from a laparoscopy.[1]

Section 3.2 | **Robotically-Assisted Systems and Augmented Reality**

WHAT ARE ROBOTICALLY-ASSISTED SURGICAL SYSTEMS?

Different computer-assisted surgical systems can be used for preoperative planning, surgical navigation, and surgical procedures. Robotically-assisted surgical (RAS) devices are one type of computer-assisted surgical system. Sometimes referred to as "robotic surgery," RAS devices enable the surgeon to use computer and software technology to control and move surgical instruments through one or more tiny incisions in the patient's body for various surgical procedures.

The benefits of RAS devices may include their ability to facilitate minimally invasive surgery and assist with complex tasks in confined areas of the body. The device is not actually a robot because it cannot perform surgery without direct human control.

[1] MedlinePlus, "Laparoscopy," National Institutes of Health (NIH), March 6, 2023. Available online. URL: https://medlineplus.gov/lab-tests/laparoscopy. Accessed April 8, 2024.

RAS devices generally have several components, which may include:

- **Console**. Where the surgeon sits during surgery. The console is the control center of the device and allows the surgeon to view the surgical field through a three-dimensional (3D) endoscope and control the movement of the surgical instruments.
- **Bedside cart**. Includes three or four hinged mechanical arms, a camera (endoscope), and surgical instruments that the surgeon controls during surgical procedures.
- **Separate cart**. Contains supporting hardware and software components, such as an electrosurgical unit (ESU), suction/irrigation pumps, and a light source for the endoscope.

Most surgeons use multiple surgical instruments and accessories with the RAS device, such as scalpels, forceps, graspers, dissectors, cautery, scissors, retractors, and suction irrigators.

COMMON USES OF ROBOTICALLY-ASSISTED SURGICAL DEVICES

The U.S. Food and Drug Administration (FDA) has cleared RAS devices for use by trained physicians in an operating room environment for laparoscopic surgical procedures in general surgery, cardiac, colorectal, gynecologic, head and neck, thoracic, and urologic surgical procedures. Some common procedures that may involve RAS devices are gallbladder removal, hysterectomy, and prostatectomy.

While RAS is safe and effective for performing certain procedures when used appropriately and with proper training, the FDA has not granted marketing authorization for any RAS device system in the United States specifically for the prevention or treatment of cancer.

RECOMMENDATIONS FOR PATIENTS ABOUT ROBOTICALLY-ASSISTED SURGERY

Robotically-assisted surgery is an important treatment option but may not be appropriate in all situations. Talk to your physician about the risks and benefits of RAS, as well as the risks and benefits of other treatment options.

Patients considering treatment with RAS should discuss the options for these devices with their health-care provider and inquire about their surgeon's training and experience with them.

RECOMMENDATIONS FOR HEALTH-CARE PROVIDERS ABOUT ROBOTICALLY-ASSISTED SURGERY

Robotically-assisted surgery is safe and effective for performing certain procedures appropriately and with proper training. The FDA regulates devices to provide reasonable assurance of their safety and effectiveness for their intended uses. For RAS devices, this includes ensuring manufacturers implement adequate training programs for both new and experienced users. The FDA does not supervise or provide accreditation for physician training nor oversees training and education related to legally marketed medical devices. Instead, the development and implementation of training is the responsibility of the manufacturer, physicians, and health-care facilities. In some cases, professional societies and specialty board certification organizations may also develop and support training for their specialty physicians.

Physicians, hospitals, and facilities that use RAS devices should ensure that surgeons are properly trained and have appropriate credentials to perform surgical procedures with these devices. Device users should also ensure they maintain their credentialing. Hospitals and facilities should also ensure that other surgical staff who use these devices complete proper training.

Users should realize there are several models of RAS devices. Each model may operate differently and not have the same functions. Users should know the differences between the models and get appropriate training on each model.

If they suspect a problem or complications associated with using RAS devices, the FDA encourages them to file a voluntary report through MedWatch: The FDA Safety Information and Adverse Event Reporting Program. Health-care personnel employed by facilities subject to the FDA's user facility reporting requirements should follow the reporting procedures established by their facilities. Prompt reporting of adverse events can help the FDA identify and better understand the risks associated with medical devices.

ROBOTICALLY-ASSISTED SURGICAL DEVICES AND CANCER

The FDA's Updated Safety Communication

The FDA has become aware of the continued use of RAS devices for the prevention of cancer and treatment of patients with cancer. Health-care providers and patients need to understand that the FDA has not granted marketing authorization for any RAS devices specifically for the prevention or treatment of cancer.

Use of Robotically-Assisted Surgical Devices in Cancer Patients

The FDA regulates medical devices but generally does not regulate the practice of medicine within a health-care practitioner-patient relationship. The FDA has evaluated and cleared RAS devices for use in certain types of surgical procedures commonly performed in patients with cancer, such as hysterectomy, prostatectomy, and colectomy. These clearances are based on short-term (30-day) patient follow-up. The safety and effectiveness of RAS devices for the prevention and treatment of cancer, based on cancer-related outcomes, such as overall survival, recurrence, and disease-free survival, have not been established.

Robotically-Assisted Surgical Devices and Mastectomy Procedures

There is little evidence on the safety and effectiveness of the use of RAS devices in patients undergoing mastectomy for the prevention or treatment of breast cancer, and the FDA has not granted any RAS device marketing authorization for mastectomy. For patients undergoing mastectomy, the surgical approach used with RAS devices differs from conventional surgical approaches. The effect of these differences on the prevention of cancer, overall survival, recurrence, and disease-free survival has not been established.

Robotically-Assisted Surgical Devices and Cervical Cancer

The FDA is aware of limited reports that conclude that minimally invasive surgery (including laparoscopic surgery or surgery using RAS devices) was associated with a lower rate of long-term survival compared with open abdominal surgery. Other reports have demonstrated no significant difference in long-term survival when these types of surgical procedures are compared. Clinicians and patients should be aware of this information when making treatment decisions.

FDA ACTIVITIES RELATED TO ROBOTICALLY-ASSISTED SURGICAL DEVICES

- **The FDA continues to receive and analyze medical device reports (MDRs) related to RAS devices.** Most reports concern device malfunctions, such as component breakage, mechanical problems, and image or display issues. Generally, these reports are not associated with injuries. However, the FDA has received reports of injuries and deaths related to RAS devices.
- **The FDA receives mandatory reports from device manufacturers, device user facilities, and importers, and voluntary reports from health-care professionals, patients, caregivers, and consumers.** These multiple sources can lead to duplications and inaccuracies. Because reports submitted to the FDA can also contain incomplete, inaccurate, or unverified information, confirming whether a device actually caused a specific event can be difficult based solely on information provided in a given report. Submitting a report to the FDA does not necessarily indicate a faulty or defective medical device.
- **The FDA also continues to evaluate information on RAS devices from other sources, such as published studies and case histories, in addition to the reports described above.** Monitoring the safety and effectiveness of medical devices relies on multiple sources of information to inform decisions about a device's safety and effectiveness.

- **To obtain additional information, the FDA conducted a small-sample Medical Product Safety Network (MedSun) survey of experienced surgeons who use RAS devices in various procedures.** The goal was to better understand the users' perspectives and the different challenges identified when using this system to perform surgery compared to conventional surgical procedures.
- **The FDA is working with professional societies to encourage training and education associated with using these devices.**
- **The FDA encourages academic and research institutions, professional societies, RAS device experts, and manufacturers to establish patient registries to gather data on the use of RAS devices for all uses, including the prevention and treatment of cancer.** Such real-world evidence may help characterize surgeons' learning curves, assess long-term clinical outcomes, and identify problems early to help enhance patient safety. However, clinical studies to determine the safety and effectiveness of RAS devices for unapproved uses such as the treatment of cancer, including when a registry infrastructure is used to collect the clinical study data, must be done under an investigational device exemption (IDE).
- **The FDA routinely monitors the postmarket performance of marketed devices and inspects manufacturing facilities that make the medical devices and will continue to collect and analyze all available information regarding RAS devices to better understand the risks and benefits.** The FDA will keep the public informed if significant new information becomes available.[1]

---

[1] "Computer-Assisted Surgical Systems," U.S. Food and Drug Administration (FDA), June 21, 2022. Available online. URL: www.fda.gov/medical-devices/surgery-devices/computer-assisted-surgical-systems. Accessed April 8, 2024.

AUGMENTED REALITY AND VIRTUAL REALITY IN MEDICAL DEVICES

What Are Augmented Reality and Virtual Reality?

Augmented reality (AR) is a real-world augmented experience that overlays or mixes simulated digital imagery with the real world as seen through a camera or display, such as a smartphone or head-mounted or heads-up display (HUD). Digital imagery may interact with real surroundings (often controlled by users). This is sometimes referred to as "mixed" or "merged reality."

Virtual reality (VR) is a virtual world immersive experience that may require a headset to completely replace a user's surrounding view with a simulated, immersive, and interactive virtual environment.

The terms extended reality, or AR and VR, are often used to encompass the two approaches. For the purposes of this web page, we will use the terms augmented reality and virtual reality.

Some real-world examples of AR and VR applications already being used to treat patients include:

- an AR system that overlays medical images onto a patient during an operation to help guide the surgeon's technique
- a VR system that is used to treat posttraumatic stress disorder (PTSD) in army veterans
- a VR rehabilitation therapy that simulates real-life situations to improve physical functions for patients who have experienced a physical disability associated with a stroke or other medical condition

How Are Augmented Reality and Virtual Reality Affecting Medical Devices?

Augmented reality/virtual reality can deliver some clinical services—normally delivered only in clinics and hospitals—to patients in their homes or other nonclinical settings. This could enable patients, including the socioeconomically vulnerable and underserved communities, the elderly or disabled, to access needed health-care services when accessing them in person would otherwise be difficult, and this could make it easier and more likely for patients to complete treatment and monitoring regimens.

There are several treatment domains in which AR and VR are used to treat patients. Among those domains are:

- pediatric diagnostics and treatments
- pain management
- mental health
- neurological disorders
- surgery planning
- intraoperative procedures
- ophthalmic diagnostics
- telemedicine
- virtual care
- postoperative and other rehabilitation therapies

Relative to current therapies, an AR/VR device may introduce new benefits and novel approaches. Such benefits may be identified across a wide variety of patients, or it may be more beneficial for some patients than others. A device may demonstrate particular benefit for underserved populations (e.g., patients with more limited access to medical care) or vulnerable populations (e.g., children, patients with mental health or cognitive impairment). However, an AR/VR device may have risks as well, including risks related to the usability of the device (such as neck pain from the weight of the headset), and risks related to the content and images that the AR/VR technologies provide (such as low contrast images, display errors such as location or depth of anatomy, information overload, dizziness, fatigue, or effects on vision).

- Examples of probable benefits:
  - increase access to necessary health-care when accessing in person would be difficult
  - improve health-care professionals' ability to prepare for certain treatments
  - fulfill unmet medical needs
  - mitigate preoperative anxiety
  - make procedures less invasive
  - accelerate diagnoses
  - allow for self-directed care

- Examples of probable risks:
  - cybersickness
  - head and neck strain
  - cybersecurity risks
  - privacy risks
  - distraction in the operating room
  - effects of AR/VR on populations
  - unknown side effects and/or risks (particularly in pediatrics or other vulnerable populations)
  - potentially worsening disparities in diagnostics and treatment[2]

Section 3.3 | Laser Technology in Modern Medicine

MEDICAL LASERS

Medical lasers use precisely focused light sources to treat or remove tissues.

How Lasers Work

The term laser stands for Light Amplification by Stimulated Emission of Radiation. Ordinary light, such as that from a light bulb, has many wavelengths and spreads in all directions. Laser light, on the other hand, has a specific wavelength. It is focused on a narrow beam, creating very high-intensity light. Because lasers can focus accurately on tiny areas, they can be used for precise surgical work or cutting through tissue (in place of a scalpel).

With proper use, lasers allow the surgeon to accomplish more complex tasks, reduce blood loss, decrease postoperative discomfort, reduce the chance of wound infection, and achieve better wound healing.

---

[2] "Augmented Reality and Virtual Reality in Medical Devices," U.S. Food and Drug Administration (FDA), November 22, 2023. Available online. URL: www.fda.gov/medical-devices/digital-health-center-excellence/augmented-reality-and-virtual-reality-medical-devices. Accessed April 8, 2024.

Risks of Laser Surgery

As with any type of surgery, laser surgery has potential risks, including incomplete treatment of the problem, pain, infection, bleeding, scarring, and skin color changes. However, laser surgery uses nonionizing radiation, so it does not have the same long-term risks as x-rays or other types of ionizing radiation.

SURGICAL PROCEDURES USING LASERS

Lasers are used in many types of surgical procedures, such as:

- **Cosmetic surgery**. Removal of tattoos, scars, stretch marks, sunspots, wrinkles, birthmarks, spider veins, or hair.
- **Refractive eye surgery**. Reshaping the cornea to correct or improve vision, as in laser-assisted in situ keratomileusis (LASIK) or photorefractive keratectomy (PRK).
- **Dental procedures**. Endodontic/periodontic procedures, tooth whitening, and oral surgery.
- **General surgery**. Tumor removal, cataract removal, breast surgery, plastic surgery, and most other surgical procedures[1]

ADVANTAGES OF LASERS

The advantages of lasers include:

- greater precision than standard surgical tools
- less damage to normal tissues
- usually less pain
- less bleeding, swelling, and scarring
- reduced operating time
- faster healing
- decreased risk of infections
- can be performed in an outpatient setting

[1] "Medical Lasers," U.S. and Drug Food Administration (FDA), August 3, 2022. Available online. URL: www.fda.gov/radiation-emitting-products/surgical-and-therapeutic-products/medical-lasers. Accessed April 8, 2024.

Patients should consult with their health-care provider about whether laser therapy is appropriate.

LIMITATIONS OF LASERS

The limitations of lasers include:

- Surgeons must have specialized training.
- Strict safety precautions must be followed.
- Laser treatment is expensive and requires bulky equipment.
- The effects of laser therapy may not last long.
- Treatment may need to be repeated for full benefit.[2]

Section 3.4 | Cryosurgery

WHAT IS CRYOSURGERY?

Cryosurgery is a treatment that uses extreme cold, produced by liquid nitrogen or argon gas, to destroy cancer cells and abnormal tissue. This local treatment is directed toward a specific part of the body and is used to treat tumors on the skin as well as certain tumors inside the body. Cryosurgery is also known as "cryotherapy" or "cryoablation."

CANCERS TREATED WITH CRYOSURGERY

Cryosurgery can be used to treat the following types of cancer:

- retinoblastoma
- skin cancers, including basal cell carcinomas (BCC) and squamous cell carcinomas (SCC)
- skin lesions from AIDS-related Kaposi sarcoma
- early-stage prostate cancer

---

[2] Surveillance, Epidemiology, and End Results (SEER) Program, "Laser Surgery," National Cancer Institute (NCI), December 21, 2023. Available online. URL: https://training.seer.cancer.gov/treatment/surgery/types/primary/specialized/laser-surgery.html. Accessed April 8, 2024.

- liver cancer confined to the liver
- bone cancer, mostly chondrosarcoma
- nonsmall cell lung cancer (NSCLC)

Cryosurgery is also used to treat noncancerous conditions, including:

- skin growths called actinic keratoses that can turn into cancer
- abnormal cell changes in the cervix that can turn into cervical cancer, known as "cervical intraepithelial neoplasia" (CIN) or "cervical precancer"
- benign bone tumors, such as enchondroma, giant cell tumor (GCT), aneurysmal bone cyst (ABC), and chondroblastoma

HOW DOES CRYOSURGERY TREAT CANCER?

Cryosurgery freezes tissue, causing cells in the treated area to die. For tumors on the skin, the doctor applies liquid nitrogen directly to the abnormal area with a cotton swab or spraying device. For tumors inside the body, the doctor may use a cryoprobe to freeze the tumor tissue. Cryoprobes may be inserted into the body during surgery or through a small cut in the skin. As liquid nitrogen or argon gas flows through the cryoprobe, the doctor places it directly on the tumor. Ultrasound or magnetic resonance imaging (MRI) guides the cryoprobe to the correct spot, helping to limit damage to nearby healthy tissue. Sometimes, more than one cryoprobe is used to freeze different parts of the tumor.

When the frozen tissue thaws, the cells die. Tumors frozen inside the body are absorbed, while tumors frozen on the skin form a scab that falls off as the damaged skin heals.

Cryosurgery may be used with other cancer treatments, such as hormone therapy, chemotherapy, immunotherapy, radiation therapy, or surgery. For example, tissue remaining after a primary bone tumor has been removed by surgery may be treated with cryotherapy to reduce the risk of recurrence.

BENEFITS OF CRYOSURGERY

Cryosurgery offers many benefits:

- For tumors inside the body, only a small cut or puncture is usually needed to insert the cryoprobe through the skin, reducing pain, bleeding, and other surgical complications.
- It can often be done with local anesthesia and may not require a hospital stay.
- As a local treatment, it allows doctors to focus on a precise area, reducing damage to nearby healthy tissue.
- It can be repeated safely and used with other cancer treatments.
- It may be an option for tumors that cannot be removed with surgery or for patients who cannot undergo surgery due to age or other medical conditions.
- It may be used when cancer does not respond to standard treatments.

DRAWBACKS OF CRYOSURGERY

Some limitations of cryosurgery include:

- uncertain long-term control of cancer or improvement in survival for some uses
- limited to treating tumors that can be seen with imaging tests
- possible lack of insurance coverage, as the long-term value of cryosurgery for some cancers and precancers is still being tested

SIDE EFFECTS OF CRYOSURGERY

Cryosurgery can cause side effects, which vary depending on the treated area:

- Treating abnormal cervical cells can cause cramping, pain, or bleeding.
- Treating skin tumors may result in scarring and swelling. If nerves are damaged, there may be a loss of feeling. Rarely, it may cause a loss of skin pigment or hair in the treated area.

- Treating tumors in bone may damage nearby bone tissue, potentially causing broken bones.
- Treating liver tumors may damage the bile ducts and major blood vessels, leading to heavy bleeding or infection.
- Treating prostate cancer can cause urine flow blockage, incontinence, impotence, and rectal damage. Side effects are more likely if radiation therapy to the prostate has also been performed.

WHERE TO GO FOR CRYOSURGERY

Simple procedures can be done in a doctor's office as an outpatient. More complex procedures may require a hospital stay. A few hospitals and cancer centers have skilled doctors and equipment for complex procedures. Consult your doctor or contact hospitals and cancer centers in your area to determine if they use cryosurgery.

RESEARCH IN CRYOSURGERY

Researchers are studying cryosurgery as a potential treatment for:

- oral cancer and conditions of the mouth that can turn into cancer
- breast cancer
- colon cancer
- pancreatic cancer
- kidney cancer

Studies are also exploring the use of cryotherapy in combination with other cancer treatments, such as hormone therapy, chemotherapy, immunotherapy, radiation therapy, and surgery.[1]

---

[1] "Cryosurgery to Treat Cancer," National Cancer Institute (NCI), June 21, 2021. Available online. URL: www.cancer.gov/about-cancer/treatment/types/surgery/cryosurgery. Accessed April 8, 2024.

Chapter 4 | Telehealth and Intraoperative Monitoring

WHAT IS TELEHEALTH?

Telehealth is broadly defined as the use of communications technologies to provide and support health care at a distance. It has become a valuable tool for improving health through advances in communications, computer science, informatics, and medical technologies. Telehealth can be as simple as two doctors discussing a patient's care over the phone or as complex as using robotic technology to perform surgery from a remote site. Today, telehealth is often associated with the remote monitoring of a patient's condition; for instance, blood pressure, heart rate, and other health measurements can be obtained by a device worn by the patient and electronically sent to medical personnel.

INTRAOPERATIVE MONITORING

Intraoperative monitoring (IOM) is a technique that allows a surgeon to continuously check, record, and test during a difficult surgical procedure. In neurological surgeries, IOM is used to detect potentially damaging changes in brain, spinal cord, and peripheral nerve function before irreversible damage occurs. Rural hospitals often lack the expertise to perform this type of monitoring. Remote IOM uses systems to transmit data, voice, and images over the Internet to a monitoring site. An expert can then inform the on-site surgeons of any issues as the surgery progresses.[1]

[1] "Telehealth," National Institute of Biomedical Imaging and Bioengineering (NIBIB), December 2019. Available online. URL: www.nibib.nih.gov/sites/default/files/Telehealth_Fact_Sheet.pdf. Accessed June 29, 2024.

INTRAOPERATIVE NEUROPHYSIOLOGICAL TESTING

Intraoperative neurophysiological testing identifies and prevents complications during surgery on the nervous system, its blood supply, or adjacent tissue. Monitoring can identify new neurologic impairment, distinguish or separate nervous system structures (e.g., around or in a tumor), and demonstrate which tracts or nerves are still functional. It provides reassurance to the surgeon that no identifiable complications have been detected up to a certain point, allowing for more thorough surgical intervention.

Some high-risk patients may only be candidates for surgery if monitoring is available.

Covered Indications

Intraoperative testing is considered reasonable and necessary for the following procedures:

- surgery of the aortic arch, its branch vessels, or thoracic aorta, including carotid artery surgery, when there is a risk of cerebral or spinal cord ischemia
- resection of epileptogenic brain tissue or tumor
- resection of brain tissue near the primary motor cortex requiring brain mapping
- protection of cranial nerves, including resection of tumors involving the cranial nerves, cavernous sinus tumors, microvascular decompression of cranial nerves, skull base surgery near cranial nerves, and surgeries of the foramen magnum
- procedures like oval or round window graft, endolymphatic shunt for Meniere disease, vestibular section for vertigo
- correction of scoliosis or spinal cord deformity involving traction of the cord
- protection of the spinal cord during surgeries near the cord or during spinal instrumentation requiring pedicle screws or distraction
- decompressive procedures on the spinal cord or cauda equina for myelopathy or claudication where spinal cord or nerve function is at risk

- spinal cord tumors and fractures with the risk of cord compression
- neuromas of peripheral nerves of the brachial plexus when there is a risk to major sensory or motor nerves
- surgery or embolization for intracranial AV malformations
- surgery for arteriovenous malformation of the spinal cord
- embolization of bronchial artery AVMs or tumors
- cerebral vascular aneurysms
- surgery for intractable movement disorders
- arteriography with test occlusion of the carotid artery
- circulatory arrest with hypothermia (excluding surgeries performed under circulatory bypass)
- distal aortic procedures with the risk of spinal cord ischemia
- leg lengthening procedures involving traction on the sciatic nerve or other nerve trunks
- basal ganglia movement disorders
- surgery resulting from traumatic injury to the spinal cord or brain
- deep brain stimulation (DBS)
- certain thyroid surgeries
    - Intraoperative neurophysiologic monitoring during thyroid surgery is considered reasonable and necessary if the monitoring service adheres to essential standards and the procedure involves high-risk total removal of a thyroid lobe, removal of the entire gland, or re-entry into a prior surgical field where scar tissue obscures the recurrent laryngeal nerve.

Limitations

Intraoperative neurophysiologic testing must be ordered by the operating surgeon and performed by a physician who is not the operating surgeon, technical/surgical assistant, or anesthesiologist. The benefits of this testing are attainable under optimal recording and interpreting conditions, including the presence of a well-trained technologist and supervision by a trained clinical neurophysiologist. Continuous communication between the surgical team and monitoring staff is essential.

Intraoperative monitoring is considered reasonable and necessary only when performed in inpatient and outpatient hospital settings or Ambulatory Surgical Centers. It is unnecessary for surgeries where historical data and current practices reveal no potential for neural damage. Monitoring from a remote site is permissible, provided a trained technician is continuously present in the operating room and real-time communication with the supervising physician is maintained.

Medicare does not reimburse "incident to" care in the hospital setting and requires exclusive undivided attention of the monitoring physician for coverage. Claims for physician services must reflect only the time devoted to monitoring. Continuous monitoring requires at least eight recording channels (16 if EEG is monitored) and real-time auditory or written communication capabilities between the supervising physician and the operating room.[2]

[2] "Intraoperative Neurophysiological Testing," Centers for Medicare & Medicaid Services (CMS), November 8, 2019. Available online. URL: www.cms.gov/medicare-coverage-database/view/lcd.aspx?LCDId=35003&DocID=L35003. Accessed June 29, 2024.

Chapter 5 | **Future Trends in Surgery**

Ever wonder what the future holds for health-care technologies? New tools are already helping surgeons get a closer look inside your body. Robots enable operations that require only a small incision. Surgery is becoming less invasive, more effective, and safer. New materials equip surgeons with better ways to reconstruct tissues and promote faster healing.

Now you can explore the tools of the future with National Institutes of Health's (NIH) new interactive app. Float through a virtual 3D operating room to learn about technologies, including new imaging tools, robotics, biomaterials, and more. As you hover, click on objects to see the tools being developed right now.

Watch a robot perform surgery. Robots can make stitches that are far tinier than a surgeon's. They can also bend and twist in ways that a surgeon's hand cannot. Click on another tool to watch foam expanding inside a blood vessel to block an aneurysm, a balloon-like bulge in danger of bursting. There are many technologies to explore.[1]

WHAT ARE IMAGE-GUIDED ROBOTIC INTERVENTIONS?

Image-guided robotic interventions are medical procedures that integrate sophisticated robotic and imaging technologies, primarily to perform minimally invasive surgery. This integrated technology offers distinct advantages for both patients and physicians.

- **Imaging**. In image-guided procedures, the surgeon is guided by images from various techniques, including

[1] *NIH News in Health*, "Explore Future Surgery Tools," National Institutes of Health (NIH), July 2017. Available online. URL: https://newsinhealth.nih.gov/2017/07/explore-future-surgery-tools. Accessed July 9, 2024.

magnetic resonance (MR) and ultrasound. Images can also be obtained using tiny cameras attached to probes that fit into a minimal incision. The camera allows the surgery to be performed using a much smaller incision than in traditional surgery.

- **Robotics**. The surgeon's hands and traditional surgical tools are too large for small incisions. Instead, thin, finger-like robotic tools are used to perform the surgery. As the surgeon watches the image on the screen, she uses a tele-manipulator to transmit and direct hand and finger movements to a robot, which can be controlled by hydraulic, electronic, or mechanical means. Robotic tools can also be controlled by computer. One advantage of a computerized system is that a surgeon could potentially perform the surgery from anywhere in the world. This type of long-distance surgery is currently in the experimental phase. The experiments illustrate the life-saving potential for such surgeries when a delicate operation requires a specially trained surgeon in a distant location.

Additionally, doctors can use image-guided robotic interventions to more accurately target tumors when performing biopsies and radiation treatments.

WHAT ARE THE ADVANTAGES OF MINIMALLY INVASIVE PROCEDURES?

Minimally invasive surgery can reduce the damage to surrounding healthy tissues, thus decreasing the need for pain medication and reducing patients' recovery time. For surgeons, image-guided interventions using robots also have the advantage of reducing fatigue during long operations, allowing the surgeon to perform the procedure while seated.

Examples of Image-Guided Robotic Interventions

- **Robotic prostatectomy**. Complete prostate removal is performed through a series of small incisions, compared with a single large incision in traditional surgery. The small incisions result in shorter postoperative recovery, less scarring, and a faster return to normal activities.

- **Ablation techniques for early cancers**. Patients with early kidney cancer can be treated with minimally invasive procedures to destroy small tumors. Cryoablation uses cold energy to destroy the tumors. Doctors use computed tomography (CT) and ultrasound imaging to position a needle-like probe within each kidney tumor. Once in position, the tip of the probe is super-cooled to encase the tumor in a ball of ice. Alternate freeze/thaw cycles kill the tumor cells. Other minimally invasive methods of destroying early kidney cancers include heating the tumor cells and surgical removal using a robotic device. Many patients can go home the same day and resume regular activities within several days.
- **Orthopedics**. Image-guided robotic procedures are improving the precision and outcome of a number of orthopedic procedures. For example, partial knee resurfacing surgeries target only the damaged sections of the knee joint. Orthopedic surgeons combine the use of a robotic surgical arm and fiber optic cameras, resulting in patients retaining more of their normal healthy tissue. Image-guided robotic procedures also improve total knee replacements, allowing precise alignment and positioning of knee implants. The result is more natural knee function, better range of motion, and improved balance for patients.

NIBIB-FUNDED RESEARCH IN IMAGE-GUIDED ROBOTIC INTERVENTIONS

- **Portable robot using 3D near-infrared imaging**. Drawing blood and inserting IV lines are common medical procedures. However, for many patients, it can be difficult to find veins and accurately insert the needle, resulting in patient injury. National Institute of Biomedical Imaging and Bioengineering (NIBIB)-funded scientists are developing a portable, lightweight medical robot to help perform these procedures. The device uses 3D near-infrared imaging to identify an appropriate vein for the robot to insert the needle. The goal is to integrate the imaging system and software into a miniaturized version of the prototype robot, resulting in a compact, low-cost system that greatly improves the safety and accuracy of accessing veins.

- **Robot-assisted needle guidance for liver tumors.** Radiofrequency ablation (RFA) is a minimally invasive treatment that kills tumors with heat and can be a life-saving option for patients who are not eligible for surgery. NIBIB-funded scientists are developing highly flexible needles that can be guided along controlled, curved paths through tissue, allowing the removal of tumors that are not accessible by a straight-line path. This technology combines needle flexibility with a 3D ultrasound guidance system, increasing accuracy and reducing damage to healthy tissue during tumor removal.
- **Swallowable capsule for Barrett esophagus.** Barrett esophagus is a precancerous condition requiring repeated biopsies. NIBIB-funded researchers are developing a swallowable, pill-sized device to improve the management and treatment of this condition. The patient swallows the pill, which is attached to a thin tether made of cable and optic fiber. The device detects microscopic areas of the esophagus that may show evidence of disease and uses a laser to collect samples—a technology known as "laser capture microdissection." The physician retrieves the device without discomfort, and the collected samples are examined for disease. This minimally invasive device improves patient comfort and provides a precise molecular profile of the biopsied regions, helping physicians better monitor and treat the disorder.[2]

[2] "Image-Guided Robotic Interventions," National Institute of Biomedical Imaging and Bioengineering (NIBIB), July 2016. Available online. URL: www.nibib.nih.gov/science-education/science-topics/image-guided-robotic-interventions. Accessed July 9, 2024.

FIBER-OPTIC "NERVES" ENABLE SENSITIVE SURGERY TOOLS

- **NASA technology**. Can you make a robot feel? That was the question posed to Johnson Space Center engineer Toby Martin. NASA wanted tactile sensing for Robonaut's hands. Intelligent Fiber Optic Systems (IFOS) Corporation, a company familiar with NASA, responded with a proposal for "optical nerves," optical fibers with reflective microstructures called "fiber Bragg gratings." These gratings change their reflective wavelength when subjected to strain or temperature changes. The technology can determine the position of each finger in real-time by measuring the strain from bending, and it can detect vibrations and textures.
- **Technology transfer**. NASA's Small Business Innovation Research (SBIR) and Small Business Technology Transfer (STTR) programs funded the development of this technology. IFOS adapted an optical chip concept for a scalable architecture, leading to a photonic spectral processor that precisely determines sensor wavelengths. The technology has multiple applications, including medical tools, which require high-resolution, multidimensional mapping.
- **Benefits**. IFOS has found many possible medical applications for its fiber-sensing technology, such as instrumented biopsy needles and MRI-guided surgical tools. The company is developing a robotic prosthetic hand that uses fiber-optic sensors and ultrasonic imaging technology to sense muscle activation in the forearm, enabling high precision control. Other projects include a "lab-on-a-chip" device for monitoring biochemical concentrations.[3]

---

[3] "Fiber-Optic 'Nerves' Enable Sensitive Surgery Tools," National Aeronautics and Space Administration (NASA), 2020. Available online. URL: https://spinoff.nasa.gov/Spinoff2020/hm_4.html. Accessed July 9, 2024.

Part 2 | **Preparing for Surgery**

Chapter 6 | What You Need to Know about Surgery

Most operations are not emergencies and are considered elective surgery. This means you have time to learn about your operation to ensure it is the best treatment for you. You also have time to work with your surgeon to make the surgery as safe as possible. Be active in your health care to receive quality care.

Your regular doctor is your primary care doctor. He or she may suggest that you have surgery and may refer you to a surgeon. You may also want to find another surgeon to get a second opinion, to confirm if surgery is the right treatment for you. You might want to ask friends or coworkers for the names of surgeons they have used.

GET THE BASIC FACTS

Why Do You Need an Operation?

There are many reasons to have surgery. Some operations can relieve or prevent pain. Others can reduce symptoms or improve body function. Some surgeries are done to diagnose a problem. Surgery can also save your life. Your doctor will tell you the purpose of the procedure. Ensure you understand how the proposed operation will help fix your medical problem. For example, if something is going to be repaired or removed, find out why it needs to be done.

What Operation Are You Recommending?

Ask your surgeon to explain the surgery and how it is done. Your surgeon can draw a picture or diagram and explain the steps of the surgery.

Is there more than one way of doing the operation? One way may require more extensive surgery than another. Some operations that once needed large incisions (cuts in the body) can now be done using much smaller incisions (laparoscopic surgery). Some surgeries require a hospital stay for one or more days. Others let you come in and go home on the same day. Ask why your surgeon wants to do the operation one way or another.

Are There Alternatives to Surgery?

Sometimes, surgery is not the only answer to a medical problem. Medicines or treatments other than surgery, such as a change in diet or special exercises, might help you just as well—or more. Ask your surgeon or primary care doctor about the benefits and risks of these other choices. You need to know as much as possible about these benefits and risks to make the best decision.

One alternative to surgery may be watchful waiting. During a watchful wait, your doctor and you check to see if your problem improves or worsens over time. If it gets worse, you may need surgery right away. If it gets better, you may be able to wait to have surgery or not have it at all.

How Much Will the Operation Cost?

Even if you have health insurance, there may be some costs for you to pay. This may depend on your choice of surgeon or hospital. Ask what your surgeon's fee is and what it covers. Surgical fees often include some visits after the operation. You will also get a bill from the hospital for your care and from the other doctors who provided care during your surgery.

Before you have the operation, call your insurance company. They can tell you how much of the costs your insurance will pay and what share you will have to pay. If you are covered by Medicare, call 800-MEDICARE (800-633-4227) to find out your share of surgery costs.

LEARN THE BENEFITS AND RISKS

What Are the Benefits of Having the Operation?

Ask your surgeon what you will gain by having the operation. For example, a hip replacement may mean that you can walk again with ease.

Ask how long the benefits will last. For some procedures, it is not unusual for the benefits to last only a short time. You may need a second operation at a later date. For other procedures, the benefits may last a lifetime.

When finding out about the benefits of the operation, be realistic. Sometimes, patients expect too much and are disappointed with the outcome or results. Ask your doctor if there is anything you can read to help you understand the procedure and its likely results.

What Are the Risks of Having the Operation?

All operations involve some risk. Therefore, you must weigh the benefits of the operation against the risks of complications or side effects.

Complications are unplanned events linked to the operation. Typical complications are infection, too much bleeding, reaction to anesthesia, or accidental injury. Some people have a greater risk of complications because of other medical conditions. There also may be side effects after the operation. Often, your surgeon can tell you what side effects to expect. For example, there may be swelling and some soreness around the incision.

There is almost always some pain with surgery. Ask your surgeon how much pain there will be and what the doctors and nurses will do to help manage the pain. Controlling the pain will help you to be more comfortable while you heal. Controlling the pain will also help you get well faster and improve the results of your operation.

What If You Do Not Have This Operation?

Based on what you learn about the benefits and risks of the operation, you might decide not to have it. Ask your surgeon what you will gain—or lose—by not having the operation now.

Where Can You Get a Second Opinion?

Getting a second opinion from another doctor is a good way to ensure that having the operation is the best choice for you. You can ask your primary care doctor for the name of another surgeon who could review your medical file. If you consult another doctor, get your records from the first doctor so your tests do not have to be repeated.

Many health insurance plans ask patients to get a second opinion before they have certain operations that are not emergencies. If your plan does not require a second opinion, you may still ask to have one. Check with your insurance company to see if they will pay for a second opinion. You should discuss your insurance questions with your health insurance company or employee benefits office. If you are eligible for Medicare, they will pay for a second opinion.

FIND OUT MORE ABOUT YOUR OPERATION

What Kind of Anesthesia Will You Need?

Anesthesia is used so that surgery can be performed without unnecessary pain. Your surgeon can tell you whether the operation calls for local, regional, or general anesthesia and why this form of anesthesia is best for your procedure.

Local anesthesia numbs only a part of your body and only for a short period. For example, when you go to the dentist, you may get a local anesthetic called "Novocain." It numbs the gum area around a tooth. Not all procedures done with local anesthesia are painless. Regional anesthesia numbs a larger portion of your body—for example, the lower part—for a few hours. In most cases, you will be awake during the operation with regional anesthesia. General anesthesia numbs your entire body. You will be asleep during the whole operation if you have general anesthesia.

Anesthesia is quite safe for most patients. It is usually given by a specialized doctor (anesthesiologist) or nurse (nurse anesthetist), both of whom are highly skilled and trained in anesthesia.

If you decide to have an operation, ask to meet with the person who will give you anesthesia. It is okay to ask what his or her qualifications are. Ask what the side effects and risks of having anesthesia are in your case. Be sure to tell him or her what medical problems you have—including allergies—and what medicines you have been taking. These medicines may affect your response to the anesthesia. Be sure to include prescription and over-the-counter (OTC) medicines, such as vitamins and supplements.

How Long Will It Take You to Recover?

Your surgeon can tell you how you might feel and what you will be able to do—or not do—the first few days, weeks, or months after surgery. Ask how long you will be in the hospital. Find out what kind of supplies, equipment, and help you will need when you go home. Knowing what to expect can help you get better faster.

Ask how long it will be before you can go back to work or start regular exercise again. You do not want to do anything that will slow your recovery. For example, lifting a 10-pound bag of potatoes may not seem too much a week after your operation, but it could be. You should follow your surgeon's advice to recover fully as soon as possible.

MAKING SURE YOUR SURGERY IS SAFE

Check with your insurance company to find out if you may choose a surgeon or hospital or if you must use ones selected by the insurer. Ask your doctor which hospital has the best care and results for your condition if you have more than one hospital. Studies show that for some types of surgery, numbers count—using a surgeon or hospital that performs more of a particular type of surgery can improve your chance of a good result.

QUESTIONS TO ASK THE SURGEON IF YOU HAVE A CHOICE OF SURGEON OR HOSPITAL

What Are Your Qualifications?

You will want to know that your surgeon is experienced and qualified to perform the operation. Many surgeons have taken special training and passed exams by a national board of surgeons. Ask if your surgeon is board certified in surgery. Some surgeons also have the letters F.A.C.S. after their name, indicating they are Fellows of the American College of Surgeons (ACS) and have passed another review by surgeons of their surgical skills.

How Much Experience Do You Have Doing This Operation?

One way to reduce the risks of surgery is to choose a surgeon who has been well-trained to do the surgery and has plenty of experience doing it. You can ask your surgeon about his or her recent record of successes and complications with this surgery. If it is easier, you can discuss the surgeon's qualifications with your primary care doctor.

At Which Hospital Will the Operation Be Done?

Most surgeons work at one or two local hospitals. Find out where your surgery will be done and how often the same operation is performed. Research shows that patients often do better when they have surgery in hospitals with more experience in the operation. Ask your doctor about the success rate at the hospitals you can choose from. The success rate is the number of patients who improve, divided by all patients having that operation at a hospital. If your surgeon suggests using a hospital with a lower success rate for your surgery, find out why.

How Long Will I Be in the Hospital?

Most patients who had surgery stayed in the hospital overnight for one or more days. Nowadays, many patients have surgery done as an outpatient in a doctor's office, a special surgical center, or a day surgery unit of a hospital. These patients have an operation and go home the same day. Outpatient surgery is less expensive because you do not have to pay to stay in a hospital room.

Ask whether your operation will be done in the hospital or an outpatient setting, and ask which is the usual way the surgery is done. If your doctor recommends that you stay overnight in the hospital (have inpatient surgery) for an operation that is usually done as outpatient surgery—or recommends outpatient surgery that is usually done as inpatient surgery—ask why. You want to be in the right place for your operation.

HAVE THE SURGEON MARK THE SURGICAL SITE

Rarely, surgeons will make mistakes and operate on the wrong body part. Several groups of surgeons urge their members to use a marking pen to show the place where they will operate. The surgeons do this by writing directly on the patient's skin on the day of surgery. Do not be afraid to ask your surgeon to do this to make your surgery safer.[1]

[1] Agency for Healthcare Research and Quality (AHRQ), "Having Surgery? What You Need to Know," U.S. Department of Health and Human Services (HHS), October 2005. Available online. URL: www.ahrq.gov/sites/default/files/wysiwyg/patients-consumers/diagnosis-treatment/surgery/questions/surgery.pdf. Accessed April 9, 2024.

Chapter 7 | Getting a Second Opinion before Surgery

A second opinion is when another doctor, in addition to your regular doctor, gives their view about your health problem and how it should be treated. Getting a second opinion can help you make a more informed decision about your care.

Medicare Part B (medical insurance) helps pay for a second opinion before surgery. When your doctor says you have a health problem that needs surgery, you have the right to:

- know and understand your treatment choices
- have another doctor review those choices with you (second opinion)
- participate in treatment decisions by making your wishes known

WHEN SHOULD YOU GET A SECOND OPINION?

If your doctor says you need surgery to diagnose or treat a health problem that is not an emergency, consider getting a second opinion. It is up to you to decide when and if you will have surgery.

Medicare does not pay for surgeries or procedures that are not medically necessary, such as cosmetic surgery. This means that Medicare would also not pay for second opinions for such surgeries or procedures.

Do not wait for a second opinion if you need emergency surgery. Some types of emergencies may require surgery right away, such as:

- acute appendicitis
- blood clots or aneurysms
- accidental injuries

PREPARING FOR YOUR SECOND OPINION

Before you visit the second doctor:

- Ask the first doctor to send your medical records to the second doctor to avoid repeating tests.
- Call the second doctor's office to ensure they have your records.
- Write down a list of questions to take with you to the appointment.
- Ask a family member or friend to accompany you to the appointment.

During your visit with the second doctor:

- Inform the doctor about the surgery your first doctor recommended.
- Mention the tests you already had.
- Ask the questions on your list and encourage your family member or friend to ask any questions they have.

Note: *The second doctor may request additional tests. Medicare will help pay for these tests, as it does for other medically necessary services.*

WHAT IF THE FIRST AND SECOND OPINIONS ARE DIFFERENT?

If the opinions differ, you may want to:

- discuss your condition further with your first doctor
- consult a third doctor (Medicare helps pay for a third opinion if the first and second opinions differ)

Getting a second or third opinion does not mean you have to change doctors. If you decide to have surgery, you will choose which doctor you want to perform the surgery.

HOW MUCH DOES MEDICARE PAY FOR A SECOND OPINION?

Medicare Part B helps pay for a second (or third) opinion and related tests, just as it helps pay for other medically necessary services.

If you have Medicare Part B and original Medicare:

- Medicare pays 80 percent of the Medicare-approved amount.
- You usually pay 20 percent of the Medicare-approved amount after you pay your yearly Medicare Part B deductible.

DO MEDICARE ADVANTAGE PLANS COVER SECOND OPINIONS?

If you have a Medicare Advantage plan, you can get a second opinion. If the first two opinions differ, your plan will help pay for a third opinion. Keep the following in mind:

- Some plans will only help pay for a second opinion if you have a referral from your primary care doctor.
- Some plans will only help pay for a second opinion from a doctor within your plan's provider network.[1]

[1] "Getting a Second Opinion before Surgery," Centers for Medicare & Medicaid Services (CMS), December 2021. Available online. URL: www.medicare.gov/Pubs/pdf/02173-Getting-a-Second-Opinion-Before-Surgery.pdf. Accessed April 8, 2024.

Chapter 8 | **Choosing the Right Hospital**

When you are sick, you may go to the closest hospital or the hospital where your doctor practices. However, research shows that some hospitals do a better job of caring for patients with certain conditions. In a life-threatening emergency, always go to the nearest hospital. Understanding your choices will help you have a more informed discussion with your doctor or other health-care providers.

BEFORE YOU GET STARTED

Make the most of your appointments with your doctor or other health-care provider to learn about your condition and health-care needs:

- Before your appointment, make a list of topics you want to discuss with your doctor or health-care provider, such as recent symptoms, drug side effects, or other general health questions. Bring this list to your appointment.
- Bring any prescription drugs, over-the-counter (OTC) drugs, vitamins, and supplements to your appointment and review them with your doctor or health-care provider.
- Take notes during your appointment. Then, repeat what the doctor or health-care provider told you. Ask any questions you may have.
- Bring along a trusted family member or friend.
- Ask if there is any written information about your condition that you can take with you.

- Call the office if you have questions when you get home.

STEPS TO CHOOSING A HOSPITAL CHECKLIST

Step 1: Learn about the Care You Need and Your Hospital Choices

- Talk to your doctors or health-care providers:
  - Find out which hospitals they work with.
  - Ask which hospitals they think provide the best care for your condition (e.g., have enough staffing, coordinate care, promote medication safety, and prevent infection).
  - Ask how well these hospitals check and improve their quality of care.
  - Ask if the hospitals participate in Medicare or the network of your Medicare Advantage plan (such as a health maintenance organization (HMO) or preferred provider organization (PPO)) or other Medicare health plan if you have one.
- Based on your condition, ask the following questions to your doctors or health-care providers:
  - Should you consider a specialty hospital, teaching hospital (usually part of a university), community hospital, or one that does research or has clinical trials related to your condition?
  - If you need a surgeon or other specialist, what is their experience and success rate in treating your condition?
  - Who will be responsible for your overall care while you are in the hospital?
  - Will you need care after leaving the hospital, and if so, what kind of care? Who will arrange this care?
  - Are there any alternatives to hospital care?

Step 2: Think about Your Personal and Financial Needs

- Check your hospital insurance coverage:
  - Do you need permission from your Medicare health plan (such as preauthorization or a referral) before you are admitted for hospital care?

  - If you need care other than emergency care, do you have to use only the network of your Medicare health plan? Do you have to use certain hospitals or see certain surgeons or specialists?
  - Do you have to pay more to use a hospital (surgeon or specialist) that does not participate in your Medicare health plan if you have one?
  - Do you need to meet certain requirements to get care after you leave the hospital?
- Think about your preferences:
  - Do you want a hospital located near family members or friends?
  - Does the hospital have convenient visiting hours and other rules that are important to you? (e.g., can a relative or someone helping with your care stay overnight in the room with you?)

Step 3: Find and Compare Hospitals Based on Your Condition and Needs

Visit Medicare's Care Compare (www.medicare.gov/care-compare) to:

- Find hospitals by name, city, state, or ZIP code.
- Check the results of patient surveys (what patients said about their hospital experience).
- Compare the results of certain measures of quality that show how well these hospitals treat patients with certain conditions.

You can also call 800-MEDICARE (800-633-4227). Teletypewriter (TTY) users can call 877-486-2048.

Search online for other sources to compare the quality of the hospitals you are considering. Some states have laws requiring hospitals to report data about the quality and cost of their care and post the data online.

Step 4: Discuss Your Hospital Options and Choose a Hospital

- Talk with family members or friends about the hospitals you are comparing.

- Talk to your doctor or health-care provider about how the hospital information you gathered applies to you.
- Considering all the previously mentioned factors, choose the hospital that is best for you.

HOSPITAL QUALITY QUICK CHECK

Here is a quick summary of what to look for when comparing hospitals. Look for a hospital that:

- has the best experience with your condition
- checks and improves the quality of its care
- performs well on measures of quality, including a national patient survey
- participates in Medicare (and your Medicare health plan if you have one)
- meets your needs in terms of location and other factors, such as visiting hours
- is covered by your Medicare health plan[1]

[1] "Guide to Choosing a Hospital," Centers for Medicare & Medicaid Services (CMS), December 2017. Available online. URL: www.medicare.gov/Pubs/pdf/10181-Guide-Choosing-Hospital.pdf. Accessed April 8, 2024.

Chapter 9 | Medicare Coverage for Surgery

Medicare generally covers services (such as lab tests, surgeries, and doctor visits) and items (such as wheelchairs and walkers) it considers medically necessary to treat a disease or condition.

FACTORS THAT MAY AFFECT MEDICARE COVERAGE

- **The law**. Federal laws describe Medicare benefits, and state laws specify the services a particular provider is licensed to give.
- **National coverage determinations**. Medicare decides if a particular item or service is covered nationally.
- **Local coverage determinations**. In each state, local companies that process Medicare claims decide if a particular item or service is medically necessary and should be covered under Medicare's rules.

Other coverage rules and policies may also apply. Medicare may cover some items and services only in certain settings or if you have certain conditions. For example, some surgeries, such as organ transplants, can only be done in specific approved hospitals. If you are in a Medicare Advantage (MA) plan or another Medicare health plan, you may have different rules, but your plan must give you at least the same coverage as Original Medicare.

WHERE CAN YOU LEARN MORE ABOUT WHAT MEDICARE COVERS?

- **Talk to your doctor**. Discuss why you need the items or services and ask if they think Medicare will cover it.

- **Visit Medicare's coverage website.** Go to www.medicare.gov/coverage to see if your test, item, or service is covered.
- **Check your "*Medicare & You*" Handbook.** This handbook provides:
  - a general list of services covered by Medicare Part A (Hospital Insurance), such as inpatient hospital stays, home health services, hospice care, and care in a skilled nursing facility
  - a general list of services covered by Medicare Part B (Medical Insurance), such as preventive services, lab tests, x-rays, doctor services, and more
  - information on getting Medicare benefits through Original Medicare, MA Plans, and Medicare drug coverage
  - general information on coinsurance and copayment amounts, yearly deductibles for Part A and B services, and other MA Plan and Medicare drug plan costs

Visit the Publications page (www.medicare.gov/publications) to read the "*Medicare & You*" handbook, or call 800-MEDICARE (800-633-4227). Teletypewriter (TTY) users can call 877-486-2048.

If there is an item or service that Medicare usually covers but your doctor, health-care provider, or supplier thinks Medicare would not cover in your specific case, they must give you a Medicare notice, like an "Advance Beneficiary Notice of Noncoverage" (ABN), and ask you to sign it. Read this notice carefully to understand your options and payment responsibilities. You will be asked if you want the items or services listed on the notice and will have to pay for them if Medicare does not cover them. The type of notice you get depends on the health-care setting and services you are getting.

HOW DO YOU FIND OUT HOW MUCH YOU WILL HAVE TO PAY IF YOU HAVE SURGERY?

For surgeries or procedures, it may be difficult to know the exact costs in advance because the amount or type of services you will need can vary, especially if complications arise.

If you are having surgery or a procedure, here is what you can do in advance to get an estimate of your share of the cost:

- **Visit Medicare's procedure price lookup**. Go to www.medicare.gov/procedure-price-lookup to compare national average costs for procedures in certain settings.
- **Ask your doctor, surgeon, or health-care provider**. Find out how much the surgery or procedure will cost, what kind of care or services you may need after your surgery or procedure, and how much you will have to pay.
- **Check your "Medicare Summary Notice" (MSN)**. Look at your last MSN to see if you have met the deductible for Part A if you expect to be admitted to the hospital or for Part B for a doctor's visit and other outpatient care. You will need to pay the deductible amounts before Medicare will start to pay. After Medicare starts to pay, you may have copayments for the care you get.
- **Check other insurance**. See if any other insurance you have, such as Medicare Supplement Insurance (Medigap), Medicaid, or an employer retiree insurance plan, will pay. If you have MA or another Medicare health plan, contact the plan for more information.
- **Call the hospital or facility and ask for the co-payment for your specific surgery or procedure**. Remember, your costs may be higher if you need other unexpected services.
- **Visit Medicare.gov for more information about how Medicare covers inpatient versus outpatient hospital services**. You can also call 800-MEDICARE (800-633-4227), or TTY users can call 877-486-2048.

HOW CAN YOU KEEP YOUR COSTS DOWN?

- **Ask about an assignment**. Ask your doctor, other health-care provider, or supplier if they accept assignments. Assignment means your doctor, provider, or supplier has signed an agreement with Medicare (or is required by law) to accept the Medicare-approved amount as full payment for covered services.

- **Check for assistance programs.** If you have limited income and resources, you might qualify for programs to help pay for some of your health and drug costs. Check your "*Medicare & You*" handbook, or visit www.medicare.gov.[1]

[1] "Learning What Medicare Covers and Your Costs," Centers for Medicare & Medicaid Services (CMS), September 2022. Available online. URL: www.medicare.gov/Pubs/pdf/11472-Learn-What-Medicare-Covers.pdf. Accessed April 9, 2024.

Chapter 10 | Advance Care Planning

During an emergency or at the end of life, you may face questions about your loved one's medical treatment and not be able to answer them. You may assume your loved ones know what you would want, but that is not always true. In one study, people guessed nearly one out of three end-of-life decisions for their loved one incorrectly.

Research shows that you are more likely to get the care you want if you have conversations about your future medical treatment and put a plan in place. It may also help your loved ones grieve more easily and feel less burden, guilt, and depression.

WHAT IS ADVANCE CARE PLANNING?

Advance care planning involves discussing and preparing for future decisions about your medical care if you become seriously ill or unable to communicate your wishes. The most important part of advance care planning is having meaningful conversations with your loved ones. Many people also choose to put their preferences in writing by completing legal documents called "advance directives."

WHAT ARE ADVANCE DIRECTIVES?

Advance directives are legal documents that provide instructions for medical care and only go into effect if you cannot communicate your own wishes.

The following are the two most common advance directives for health care:

- **Living will**. This legal document tells doctors how you want to be treated if you cannot decide about

emergency treatment. In a living will, you can specify which common medical treatments or care you would want, which ones you would want to avoid, and under which conditions each of your choices applies.
- **Durable power of attorney for health care**. This legal document names your health-care proxy, a person who can make health-care decisions for you if you cannot communicate these yourself. Your proxy, a representative, surrogate, or agent, should know your values and wishes. A proxy can be chosen in addition to or instead of a living will. Having a health-care proxy helps you plan for situations that cannot be foreseen, such as a serious car accident or stroke.

Consider your advance directives as living documents that you review at least once yearly and update if a major life event occurs, such as retirement, moving out of state, or a significant change in your health.

WHO NEEDS AN ADVANCE CARE PLAN?

Advance care planning is not just for people who are very old or ill. At any age, a medical crisis could leave you unable to communicate your health-care decisions. Planning now for your future health care can help ensure you get the medical care you want and that someone you trust will be there to make decisions for you.

WHAT HAPPENS IF YOU DO NOT HAVE AN ADVANCE DIRECTIVE?

If you do not have an advance directive and cannot make decisions on your own, the laws of the state where you live will determine who may make medical decisions on your behalf. This is typically your spouse, your parents if they are available, or your children if they are adults. If you are unmarried and have not named your partner as your proxy, it is possible they could be excluded from decision-making. If you have no family, some states allow a close friend familiar with your values to help, or they may assign a physician to represent your best interests. To find out the laws in your state, contact your state legal aid office or state bar association.

WILL AN ADVANCE DIRECTIVE GUARANTEE THAT YOUR WISHES ARE FOLLOWED?

An advance directive is legally recognized but not legally binding. This means that your health-care provider and proxy will do their best to respect your advance directives, but there may be circumstances in which they cannot follow your wishes exactly. For example, you may be in a complex medical situation where it is unclear what you would want. This is another key reason why having conversations about your preferences is so important. Talking with your loved ones beforehand may help them better navigate unanticipated issues.

There is the possibility that a health-care provider refuses to follow your advance directives. This might happen if the decision goes against the:

- health-care provider's conscience
- health-care institution's policy
- accepted health-care standards

In these situations, the health-care provider must inform your health-care proxy immediately and consider transferring your care to another provider.

OTHER ADVANCE CARE PLANNING FORMS AND ORDERS

You might want to prepare documents to express your wishes about a single medical issue or something else not already covered in your advance directives, such as an emergency. For these types of situations, you can talk with a doctor about establishing the following orders:

- **Do-Not-Resuscitate (DNR) order**. A DNR order becomes part of your medical chart to inform medical staff in a hospital or nursing facility that you do not want cardiopulmonary resuscitation (CPR) or other life-support measures to be attempted if your heartbeat and breathing stop. Sometimes, this document is referred to as a "do-not-attempt-resuscitation" (DNAR) order or an allow natural death (AND) order. Even though a living will state that CPR is not wanted, it is helpful to have a DNR order as part of your medical file if you go to a hospital. Posting a DNR order next to your hospital bed might avoid confusion in an emergency. Without a DNR order, medical staff will attempt every effort to restore your breathing and the normal rhythm of your heart.

- **Do-Not-Intubate (DNI) order**. A similar document, a DNI order, informs medical staff in a hospital or nursing facility that you do not want to be on a ventilator.
- **Do-Not-Hospitalize (DNH) order**. A DNH order indicates to long-term care providers, such as nursing home staff, that you prefer not to be sent to a hospital for treatment at the end of life.
- **Out-of-Hospital DNR order**. An out-of-hospital DNR order alerts emergency medical personnel to your wishes regarding measures to restore your heartbeat or breathing if you are not in a hospital.
- **Physician Orders for Life-Sustaining Treatment (POLST) and Medical Orders for Life-Sustaining Treatment (MOLST) forms**. These forms provide guidance about your medical care that health-care professionals can act on immediately in an emergency. They serve as a medical order in addition to your advance directive. Typically, you create a POLST or MOLST form when you are near the end of life or critically ill and understand the specific decisions that might need to be made on your behalf. These forms may also be called "portable medical orders" or "physician orders" for scope of treatment (POST). Check with your state health department to find out if these forms are available where you live.

You may also want to document your wishes about organ, tissue, and brain donation. Additionally, learning about care options such as palliative and hospice care can help you plan ahead.

HOW CAN YOU GET STARTED WITH ADVANCE CARE PLANNING?

To get started with advance care planning, consider the following steps:

- **Reflect on your values and wishes**. This can help you think through what matters most at the end of life and guide your decisions about future care and medical treatment.
- **Talk with your doctor about advance directives**. Advance care planning is covered by Medicare as part of your annual wellness visit. If you have private health insurance, check with your insurance provider. Talking to a health-care provider can help you learn about your current health and the decisions that will likely arise. For example, you might ask about the decisions you may face if your high blood pressure leads to a stroke.
- **Choose someone you trust to make medical decisions for you**. Whether it is a family member, a loved one, or your lawyer, it is important to choose someone you trust as your health-care proxy. Once you have decided, discuss your values and preferences with them. If you are not ready to discuss specific treatments or care decisions yet, try talking about your general preferences. You can also try other ways to share your wishes, such as writing a letter or watching a video together.
- **Complete your advance directive forms**. To make your care and treatment decisions official, you can complete a living will. Similarly, once you decide on your health-care proxy, you can make it official by completing a durable power of attorney for health care.
- **Share your forms with your health-care proxy, doctors, and loved ones**. After you have completed your advance directives, make copies and store them in a safe place. Give copies to your health-care proxy,

health-care providers, and lawyer. Some states have registries that can store your advance directive for quick access by health-care providers and your proxy.
- **Keep the conversation going.** Continue to talk about your wishes and update your forms at least once each year or after major life changes. If you update your forms and files and keep your previous versions. Note the date the older copy was replaced by a new one. If you use a registry, ensure the latest version is on record.

Everyone approaches the process differently. Remember to be flexible and take it one step at a time. For example, try talking with your loved ones about what you appreciate and enjoy most about life. Your values, treatment preferences, and the people you involve in your plan may change. The most important part is to start the conversation.

HOW CAN YOU FIND ADVANCE DIRECTIVE FORMS?

You can establish your advance directives for little or no cost. Many states have their own forms that you can access and complete for free. The following are some ways you might find free advance directive forms in your state:

- **Contact your State Attorney General's office.**
- **Contact your local Area Agency on Aging (AAA).** You can find your area agency phone number by visiting the Eldercare Locator (https://eldercare.acl.gov/Public/Index.aspx) or by calling 800-677-1116.
- **Download your state's form online from national organizations.** The American Association of Retired Persons (AARP), the American Bar Association (ABA), or the National Hospice and Palliative Care Organization (NHPCO).
- **Veterans.** Contact your local Veterans Affairs (VA) office (www.va.gov/contact-us/#contact-your-local-va-facility). The VA office offers an advance directive specifically for veterans.

If you spend a lot of time in more than one state, consider preparing advance directives using the form for each state and keep a copy in each place.

Some organizations enable you to create, download, and print your forms online, but they may charge fees. Before you pay, remember there are several ways to get your forms for free. The following are some free online resources:

- **PREPARE for Your Care**. An interactive online program funded in part by the National Institute on Aging (NIA; https://prepareforyourcare.org). It is available in English and Spanish.
- **The Conversation Project**. A series of online conversation guides and advance care documents available in English, Spanish, and Chinese. The Conversation Project is a public engagement initiative led by the Institute for Healthcare Improvement (IHI; https://theconversationproject.org).

If you use forms from a website, check to ensure they are legally recognized in your state. You should also ensure the website is secure and will protect your personal information. Read the website's privacy policy and check that the website link begins with "https://" (make sure it has an "s") and also has a "small lock icon" next to its web address.

Some people also carry a card (e.g., from the American Hospital Association (AHA)) in their wallet, indicating their advance directive and where it is kept.[1]

[1] National Institute on Aging (NIA), "Advance Care Planning: Advance Directives for Health Care," National Institutes of Health (NIH), October 31, 2022. Available online. URL: www.nia.nih.gov/health/advance-care-planning-advance-directives-health-care. Accessed April 8, 2024.

Chapter 11 | Evaluating Routine Preoperative Testing

ROLE OF ROUTINE PREOPERATIVE TESTING

Traditionally, preoperative testing has been part of the preoperative care process to inform patient selection by determining fitness for anesthesia and identifying patients at high risk of postoperative complications. Routine preoperative tests, as defined by the American Society of Anesthesiologists, include a panel of blood tests, urine tests, chest radiography, and an electrocardiogram (ECG or EKG) done in the absence of any specific clinical indication or purpose. These tests are performed to identify latent abnormalities, such as anemia or silent heart disease, that could affect the planned surgical procedure and concomitant anesthesia.

EFFICACY AND COST OF ROUTINE PREOPERATIVE TESTING

Many hospitals mandate a series of laboratory tests before any operative procedure under the assumption that more information enhances patient safety and reduces liability for adverse events. However, over the past three decades, the value of routine preoperative testing has been questioned. Academic publications have identified significant costs associated with testing, estimated at $18 billion annually in the United States, without substantial patient benefits. Nonselective preoperative testing can lead to false-positive or borderline results, causing unnecessary investigations, psychological and economic burdens, postponed surgeries, and even morbidity and mortality from unnecessary evaluations, such as biopsies following false-positive results.

It remains unclear whether the benefits of true-positive test results outweigh the harms of false-positive results and the resource utilization required for testing. An alternative approach to routine preoperative testing might involve conducting a thorough history and physical examination, with selective testing based on clinical findings. However, the relative effect on patient and surgical outcomes, as well as resource utilization, of these two approaches is unknown.

VARIABILITY IN PATIENTS AND PROCEDURES

Patients undergoing surgery exhibit considerable variation in demographics, health status, comorbidities, surgical indications, and planned anesthesia types. These differences may influence the benefits of identifying abnormalities (e.g., anemia) and the potential harms of testing (e.g., delayed surgery or unnecessary procedures). Thus, it is crucial to evaluate the benefits and harms of preoperative testing in the context of specific patient and surgical factors.

IMPLEMENTATION OF PREOPERATIVE TESTING

The implementation of preoperative testing varies significantly. For some procedures, testing may be routine, such as in cataract surgeries where all patients undergo testing. Other times, testing follows a protocol, performed only if patients meet certain criteria, such as age or cardiovascular history. Elective testing, based on the clinician's individualized assessment of the patient's medical history and risks, differs from routine testing.

Inefficiencies in preoperative testing processes or failures in the handoff of test results among primary care physicians, surgeons, and anesthesiologists can affect the clinical utility of testing. Different hospitals and clinicians follow different protocols, including elective testing by the surgeon or anesthesiologist, referral to primary care physicians for testing at their discretion, and dedicated clinics with standardized protocols based on patient health and planned surgery. This variability raises questions about whether elective testing results in underutilization or overutilization of tests and whether different disciplines or clinicians' follow-ups have equivalent clinical utility.

TIMING OF PREOPERATIVE TESTS

The timing of preoperative tests is another critical factor. Hospitals or surgical centers may require testing within a specific period before surgery, such as 30 days or six months. This can lead to changes in surgical practices, like performing a second eye cataract surgery earlier to avoid repeating tests. However, there is no clear evidence supporting any particular time threshold for preoperative tests.

NEED FOR SYSTEMATIC REVIEW AND GUIDELINES

Three professional medical associations have called for a systematic review of routine preoperative testing due to wide variations in clinical practice and the need for guidelines. Such a review would have a broad clinical effect, particularly if it includes the most commonly ordered tests for both healthy patients and those with comorbidities undergoing various high- and low-risk surgeries.

Although the National Institute for Health and Clinical Excellence (NICE) in the United Kingdom published a guideline on routine preoperative tests for elective surgery in 2003, no recent comprehensive systematic reviews, including those by the Agency for Healthcare Research and Quality (AHRQ), have been conducted on this topic. The American College of Cardiology and the American Heart Association's 2007 guideline on perioperative cardiovascular evaluation partially covered routine preoperative tests but was narrower in scope.

ASSESSING THE CLINICAL UTILITY OF PREOPERATIVE TESTING

The effects of preoperative testing on patient outcomes are both direct and indirect. Direct effects include emotional and cognitive changes from testing and its results, harms associated with testing procedures (e.g., pain, hemorrhage, exposure to ionizing radiation, risk of contrast-induced nephropathy), and patient costs (time or copayments). Indirect effects include:

- **Influence on treatment choices**. Test results can influence surgical decisions and patient outcomes (e.g., increased surgical mortality risk leading to canceled surgery).

- **Prolonged time to treatment**. Testing can delay treatment for logistical reasons, either appropriately for further evaluation or unnecessarily.
- **Cascade testing**. Aberrant test results may lead to further testing, which can be appropriate if signaling a real abnormality or unnecessary if not clinically significant.

The testing volume affects resource utilization and costs, potentially overloading resources and increasing overhead. The effects of alternative testing strategies on resource utilization can be studied through cluster randomized studies or interrupted time series.[1]

[1] Effective Health Care Program, "Routine Preoperative Testing: Comparative Effectiveness Review," Agency for Healthcare Research and Quality (AHRQ), December 2019. Available online. URL: https://effectivehealthcare.ahrq.gov/products/preoperative-testing/research-protocol. Accessed July 10, 2024.

Chapter 12 | Ambulatory Surgeries

WHAT ARE AMBULATORY SURGERIES?

Surgical procedures that do not require an overnight hospital stay are ambulatory surgeries. Whether you call it outpatient surgery, ambulatory surgery, office surgery, or same-day surgery, it means the same thing.

Patients and their family members or friends are important members of the care team. The care team also includes doctors, nurses, and other health-care professionals who help take care of you. Your role in the care team is to learn about your surgery—how to prepare, what will happen, and what to expect afterward. If you have questions, ask! Speaking up if you are concerned about anything is one of the things you can do to stay safe.

PREPARING FOR YOUR SURGERY

Before any surgical procedure, your doctor might ask you to take certain steps to get ready for surgery. Here are some tips to make sure you are prepared:

- **Medical instructions**. Talk with your doctor about your medications well before your surgery. Your doctor may want to stop or change some medications, such as blood thinners, for a short time or may even want you to see another doctor before surgery. Your doctor's office will give you instructions to follow in the days before surgery. These instructions usually explain whether you need to stop medications or fill new prescriptions, when to stop eating and drinking before surgery, and other instructions. Be sure to follow all directions carefully. If you are confused about anything, call your doctor's office and ask questions.

- **Medication and allergy list.** Prepare an up-to-date list of your current medications and any allergies, and bring it with you on the day of surgery.
- **Preventing infection.** Your doctor may give you a prescription for an antibiotic to take before your surgery to help prevent infection. Be sure to fill any prescriptions before surgery and follow directions as prescribed. Do not wear deodorant, lotion, or perfume on the day of your surgery. Your doctor may also ask you to bathe with antibacterial soap or solution.
- **Shaving.** Do not shave the area where you will have the surgery. If hair needs to be removed from the operating site, your care team will do this on the day of the surgery.
- **Tobacco and alcohol.** Do not use tobacco or drink alcohol for at least 24 hours before your surgery.
- **Fasting.** Ask your doctor how long you should go without eating or drinking before your surgery.
- **Personal items.** Be prepared to remove dentures, hearing aids, glasses, contact lenses, jewelry, and hair accessories. Leave them at home if you can. If you must wear them, bring a case to put them in during surgery. Leave jewelry at home if you are concerned about losing it.
- **Support person.** Arrange to have someone, such as a family member or a trusted friend, go with you to the surgery center. This person will need to talk with the doctor after your surgery. Many medications used to keep you comfortable during surgery will affect your memory in the hours after surgery. Your support person can make sure you do not miss any important information, such as results and instructions.
- **Transportation.** Be sure someone is able to take you home after surgery. You may not be allowed to have the surgery unless you bring someone with you who can take you home.

- **Documents**. You may want to complete and sign an advance directive and health-care proxy before surgery. These documents are available on the Internet and from hospitals and many medical offices. If you prepare these, be sure to bring copies with you to the surgery center.
- **Personal information**. On the day of the surgery, make sure you bring your photo ID and health insurance information with you.

WHAT TO EXPECT ON THE DAY OF YOUR SURGERY

- **Admission**. When you arrive, you will check in with your photo ID and insurance information.
- **Preoperative area**. When it is your turn, you will move to a preoperative area. That is where a nurse will prepare you for surgery. The anesthesia provider, your doctor, and other members of your care team may talk with you during this time.
- **Staying safe**. Your care team will take steps to make sure your surgery is as safe as possible. For example, you might see a nurse using a surgical checklist or you may be asked more than once to verify what kind of surgery you are having and where on your body the surgery will be done. All members of your care team—including your support person or family members—should clean their hands. This can help keep you safe from surgical infections and other complications.

WHAT TO EXPECT AFTER THE SURGERY

- **Recovery**. After your procedure, you will probably be taken to a recovery area. There, your care team can monitor your condition to ensure your recovery is going well.
- **Talking with your surgeon or nurse**. Before you leave the recovery area, you and your support person should have the opportunity to ask questions. You may want to

know about how the surgery went or who to call in case of questions. You should have a clear understanding of what you need to do in the recovery period and whether you will need help from others.

- **Discharge**. You will be discharged to go home after you have recovered from the anesthesia. Your vital signs should be stable, and any pain or nausea should be under control. You will likely be required to have someone drive you home. You will receive written instructions on what to do at home. These instructions may include things like a medication schedule, things to avoid (such as certain activities or foods), possible complications to look out for, when to follow up with your doctor, and a number to call in case of problems.[1]

[1] Agency for Healthcare Research and Quality (AHRQ), "Getting Ready for Your Ambulatory Surgery," U.S. Department of Health and Human Services (HHS), August 2017. Available online. URL: www.ahrq.gov/hai/tools/ambulatory-surgery/sections/implementation/training-tools/getting-ready.html. Accessed April 9, 2024.

Chapter 13 | **Ensuring Patient Safety**

Chapter Contents

Section 13.1 | Tips for Safer Health Care and Preventing Medical Errors

Medical errors can occur anywhere in the health-care system: hospitals, clinics, surgery centers, doctors' offices, nursing homes, pharmacies, and patients' homes. Errors can involve medicines, surgery, diagnosis, equipment, or lab reports. These tips can help you get safer care.

STAYING SAFE

The best way to prevent errors is to be an active member of your health-care team. That means taking part in every decision about your health care. Research shows that patients who are more involved with their care tend to get better results.

MEDICINES

- Ensure all your doctors know about every medicine you are taking, including prescription and over-the-counter (OTC) medicines and dietary supplements, such as vitamins and herbs.
- Bring all your medicines and supplements to your doctor's visits. This will help your doctor review them and check for problems.
- Inform your doctor about any allergies and adverse reactions to medicines to avoid being prescribed something harmful.
- When your doctor writes a prescription, ensure you can read it. If you cannot read your doctor's handwriting, your pharmacist might be unable to either.
- Ask for information about your medicines in terms you can understand—both when your medicines are prescribed and when you get them:
  - What is the medicine for?
  - How am I supposed to take it, and for how long?
  - What side effects are likely? What do I do if they occur?

- Is this medicine safe to take with other medicines or dietary supplements I am taking?
- What food, drink, or activities should I avoid while taking this medicine?
- When picking up your medicine from the pharmacy, verify that it is the medicine your doctor prescribed.
- If you have any questions about the directions on your medicine labels, ask. For example, ask if "four times daily" means taking a dose every six hours around the clock or just during regular waking hours.
- Ask your pharmacist for the best device to measure your liquid medicine. Special devices, such as marked syringes, help people measure the right dose.
- Request written information about the side effects your medicine could cause. Knowing what might happen prepares you for potential side effects.

HOSPITAL STAYS

- **If you are in a hospital, consider asking all health-care workers who will touch you whether they have washed their hands.** Handwashing can prevent the spread of infections in hospitals.
- **When being discharged from the hospital, ask your doctor to explain the treatment plan you will follow at home.** This includes learning about your new medicines, scheduling follow-up appointments, and understanding when to resume regular activities. Ensure you know whether to continue any pre-hospital medicines. Clear instructions may prevent an unexpected return trip to the hospital.

SURGERY

- **If you are having surgery, make sure you, your doctor, and your surgeon agree on exactly what will be done.** Wrong-site surgery, though rare, is 100 percent preventable. Surgeons are expected to sign their initials directly on the site to be operated on before the surgery.

- **If you have a choice, choose a hospital where many patients have had the procedure or surgery you need.** Patients tend to have better results in hospitals experienced with their condition.

OTHER STEPS

- **Speak up if you have questions or concerns.** You have the right to question anyone involved in your care.
- **Ensure someone, such as your primary care doctor, coordinates your care.** This is especially important if you have many health problems or are hospitalized.
- **Make sure all your doctors have your important health information.** Do not assume everyone has all the information they need.
- **Ask a family member or friend to accompany you to appointments.** Even if you do not need help now, you might need it later.
- **Know that "more" is not always better.** Find out why a test or treatment is needed and how it can help you.
- **If you have a test, do not assume that no news is good news.** Ask how and when you will get the results.
- **Learn about your condition and treatments by asking your doctor and nurse and using other reliable sources.** For example, treatment options based on the latest scientific evidence are available from the Effective Health Care (EHC) website (https://effectivehealthcare.ahrq.gov/products). Ask your doctor if your treatment is based on the latest evidence.[1]

[1] Agency for Healthcare Research and Quality (AHRQ), "20 Tips to Help Prevent Medical Errors: Patient Fact Sheet," U.S. Department of Health and Human Services (HHS), November 2020. Available online. URL: www.ahrq.gov/questions/resources/20-tips.html. Accessed April 9, 2024.

Section 13.2 | Preventing Wrong-Site, Wrong-Procedure, and Wrong-Patient Errors

Few medical errors are as vivid and terrifying as those involving patients who have undergone surgery on the wrong body part, undergone the incorrect procedure, or had a procedure intended for another patient. These wrong-site, wrong-procedure, wrong-patient errors (WSPEs) are rightly termed "never events"—errors that should never occur and indicate serious underlying safety problems.

EXAMPLES OF WRONG-SITE SURGERIES

Wrong-site surgery may involve operating on the wrong side, as in the case of a patient who had the right side of her vulva removed when the cancerous lesion was on the left, or the incorrect body site. One example of surgery on the incorrect site is operating on the wrong level of the spine, a surprisingly common issue for neurosurgeons. A classic case of wrong-patient surgery involved a patient who underwent a cardiac procedure intended for another patient with a similar last name.

INCIDENCE AND PUBLICITY

While these high-profile cases of WSPEs have received much publicity, these errors are relatively rare. One study using the U.S. Department of Veterans Affairs (VA) data found that fully half of WSPEs occurred during procedures outside the operating room.

PREVENTIVE MEASURES FOR WRONG-SITE, WRONG-PROCEDURE, AND WRONG-PATIENT ERRORS

Early Efforts and Challenges

Early efforts to prevent WSPEs focused on developing redundant mechanisms for identifying the correct site, procedure, and patient, such as "sign your site" initiatives, which instructed surgeons to mark the operative site unambiguously. However, even this seemingly simple intervention proved problematic. An analysis of efforts in the United Kingdom to prevent WSPEs found that, although dissemination of a site-marking protocol increased preoperative site marking, implementation and adherence to the protocol differed significantly across surgical specialties and hospitals. Many clinicians voiced concerns about the unintended consequences of the protocol. In some cases, there was even confusion over whether the marked site indicated the area to be operated on or the area to be avoided. Despite these challenges, site marking remains a core component of the Joint Commission's Universal Protocol to prevent WSPEs.

The Role of Communication

Root cause analyses of WSPEs consistently reveal communication issues as a prominent underlying factor. The concept of the surgical time-out—a planned pause before beginning the procedure to review important aspects of the procedure with all involved personnel—was developed to improve communication in the operating room and prevent WSPEs. The Universal Protocol also specifies the use of a time-out before all procedures. Although initially designed for operating room procedures, time-outs are required before any invasive procedure. Comprehensive efforts to improve surgical safety have incorporated time-out principles into surgical safety checklists. While these checklists have been proven to improve surgical and postoperative safety, the low baseline incidence of WSPEs makes it difficult to establish that a single intervention can reduce or eliminate WSPEs.

CHALLENGES IN PREVENTION

Many cases of WSPEs would still occur despite full adherence to the Universal Protocol. Errors may happen well before the patient reaches the operating room; a time-out may be rushed or otherwise ineffective, and production pressures may contribute to errors during the procedure. Ultimately, preventing WSPEs depends on combining system solutions, strong teamwork and safety culture, and individual vigilance.

CURRENT CONTEXT

Wrong-patient, wrong-site, and wrong-procedure errors are all never considered events by the National Quality Forum (NQF) and are considered sentinel events by the Joint Commission. In February 2009, the Centers for Medicare & Medicaid Services (CMS) announced that hospitals would not be reimbursed for any costs associated with WSPEs. CMS has not reimbursed hospitals for additional costs associated with many preventable errors since 2007.[1]

INCIDENCE AND REDUCTION OF WRONG-SITE, WRONG-PROCEDURE, AND WRONG-PATIENT ERRORS IN FRANCE

A retrospective analysis of medical liability claims data examined the incidence of WSPEs in France between 2007 and 2017. Key findings include:

- WSPEs accounted for 0.4 percent of all claims during this 10-year period.
- Procedures on the wrong organ were most common, comprising 44 percent of the incidents.
- Errors involving the wrong side of the body occurred in 39 percent of the cases.
- Thirteen percent of WSPEs involved procedures performed on the wrong person.
- Wrong procedures were the least common, making up 4 percent of the cases.

The researchers found that the average number of WSPEs decreased after implementing a surgical checklist (https://psnet.ahrq.gov/issue/surgical-checklists-systematic-review-impacts-and-implementation).[2]

---

[1] Agency for Healthcare Research and Quality (AHRQ), "Wrong-Site, Wrong-Procedure, and Wrong-Patient Surgery," U.S. Department of Health and Human Services (HHS), September 7, 2019. Available online. URL: https://psnet.ahrq.gov/primer/wrong-site-wrong-procedure-and-wrong-patient-surgery. Accessed July 10, 2024.

[2] Agency for Healthcare Research and Quality (AHRQ), "Insurance Claims for Wrong-Side, Wrong-Organ, Wrong-Procedure, or Wrong-Person Surgical Errors: A Retrospective Study for 10 Years," U.S. Department of Health and Human Services (HHS), February 8, 2023. Available online. URL: https://psnet.ahrq.gov/issue/insurance-claims-wrong-side-wrong-organ-wrong-procedure-or-wrong-person-surgical-errors. Accessed July 10, 2024.

Section 13.3 | Understanding and Preventing Serious Reportable Events

NEVER EVENTS

The term "Never Event" was first introduced in 2001 by Ken Kizer, MD, former CEO of the National Quality Forum (NQF), about particularly shocking medical errors—such as wrong-site surgery—that should never occur. Over time, the term's use has expanded to signify adverse events that are unambiguous (clearly identifiable and measurable), serious (resulting in death or significant disability), and usually preventable. Since the initial Never Event list was developed in 2002, it has been revised multiple times and now consists of 29 "serious reportable events" grouped into seven categories:

- surgical or procedural events
- product or device events
- patient protection events
- care management events
- environmental events
- radiologic events
- criminal events

Serious Reportable Events in Surgical or Procedural Events

The following are some serious reportable events:

- surgery or other invasive procedure performed on the wrong body part
- surgery or other invasive procedure performed on the wrong patient
- wrong surgical or other invasive procedure performed on a patient
- unintended retention of a foreign object in a patient after surgery or other procedure
- intraoperative or immediately postoperative/postprocedural death

Most Never Events are very rare. For example, a 2006 study estimated that a typical hospital might experience a case of wrong-site surgery once every 5–10 years. However, when Never Events occur, they are devastating to patients—71 percent of events reported to the Joint Commission over the past 12 years were fatal—and may indicate a fundamental safety problem within an organization. Although individual events are uncommon, on a population basis, many patients still experience these serious errors. A 2013 study estimated that more than 4000 surgical Never Events occur yearly in the United States.

Increasing Accountability and Improving the Quality of Care

Because Never Events are devastating and preventable, health-care organizations are under increasing pressure to eliminate them completely. The Centers for Medicare & Medicaid Services (CMS) announced in August 2007 that Medicare would no longer pay for additional costs associated with preventable errors, including those considered Never Events. Since then, many states and private insurers have adopted similar policies. Since February 2009, CMS has not paid for any costs associated with wrong-site surgeries.

Never Events are also being publicly reported to increase accountability and improve the quality of care. Since the NQF disseminated its original Never Events list in 2002, 11 states have mandated reporting of these incidents whenever they occur, and an additional 16 states mandate reporting of serious adverse events (including many of the NQF Never Events). Health-care facilities are accountable for correcting systematic problems that contributed to the event, with some states (such as Minnesota) mandating the performance of a root cause analysis and reporting its results.[1]

MEDICAL HARM AND ADVERSE EVENTS

The concept of medical harm has existed since antiquity, famously discussed by Hippocrates and passed on in the word iatrogenesis, from the Greek for "originating from a physician." Since then, the topic has received attention from notable physicians. A paper in the New England Journal of Medicine (NEJM) in 1956 discussed the

[1] Agency for Healthcare Research and Quality (AHRQ), "Never Events," U.S. Department of Health and Human Services (HHS), September 7, 2019. Available online. URL: https://psnet.ahrq.gov/primer/never-events. Accessed April 8, 2024.

topic of diseases of medical progress, and this paper evolved into a book that used the phrase "iatrogenic disease" in its title.

"Adverse events" refer to harm from medical care rather than an underlying disease. Important subcategories of adverse events include:

- **Preventable adverse events**. Those that occurred due to error or failure to apply an accepted strategy for prevention.
- **Ameliorable adverse events**. Events that, while not preventable, could have been less harmful if care had been different.
- **Adverse events due to negligence**. Those occurred due to care that falls below the standards expected of clinicians in the community.

Two other terms that define hazards to patients but do not result in harm:

- **Near miss**. An unsafe situation that is indistinguishable from a preventable adverse event except for the outcome. A patient is exposed to a hazardous situation but does not experience harm through luck or early detection.
- **Error**. A broader term referring to any act of commission (doing something wrong) or omission (failing to do the right thing) that exposes patients to a potentially hazardous situation.[2]

Section 13.4 | Preventing Health-Care-Associated Infections

THE IMPORTANCE OF PREVENTING HEALTH-CARE-ASSOCIATED INFECTIONS

Did you know you can get infections in health-care settings while being treated for something else? Health-care-associated infections (HAIs)

[2] Agency for Healthcare Research and Quality (AHRQ), "Adverse Events, Near Misses, and Errors," U.S. Department of Health and Human Services (HHS), September 7, 2019. Available online. URL: https://psnet.ahrq.gov/primer/adverse-events-near-misses-and-errors. Accessed April 8, 2024.

can spread from person to person through hands, medical equipment, and more. HAIs are becoming more resistant to antibiotics and antifungals, making them difficult, and sometimes impossible, to treat.

Patients and their loved ones can help prevent HAIs, including those caused by antimicrobial-resistant germs. These tips describe how to be a safe patient and help reduce your risk of infections.

TIPS FOR PATIENT SAFETY

Communicate with Health-Care Providers

- Tell your health-care provider about any recent care, including hospitalizations in another facility or outside the United States in the last six months.
- Inform your provider if you have ever had an antimicrobial-resistant infection.
- Speak up about any questions or worries. Ask what your provider is doing to protect you.
- Report any signs of infection or if an infection is not getting better or is getting worse. Ask, "Could this be sepsis?"
- If you have a urinary or central line catheter, ask daily when it can be removed. Leaving a catheter in place too long increases the chances of infection.
- Know the signs and symptoms of infection. Skin infections usually appear as redness, pain, or drainage at the IV catheter site or surgery site and often come with a fever.
- Insist that your health-care providers never reuse a needle or syringe on more than one patient.
- Tell your health-care provider if you have three or more diarrhea episodes in 24 hours, especially if you have been taking an antibiotic.

Take Antibiotics Exactly as Prescribed

- Only take antibiotics when your provider thinks you need them.
- If prescribed antibiotics, ask if they are necessary.
- Follow all instructions given for taking them.

- Report any side effects, such as diarrhea, to your health-care provider.

Remind Everyone to Clean Their Hands

- Cleaning hands often prevents the spread of germs, including resistant germs.
- People should clean their hands every time they enter your room, before and after they touch equipment, you, or your wounds. This includes your health-care providers and visitors such as family and friends.
- Ask questions such as, "Before you start the exam, would you mind cleaning your hands again?" and "Can you clean your hands before changing my bandages?"

Allow People to Clean Your Room

- It is important to have a clean room while you are in the hospital or other health-care setting. Even if it is inconvenient, let staff clean your room.

Know When and Why Health-Care Staff Wear Gowns and Gloves

- Health-care workers may wear gowns and gloves to prevent spreading germs with their hands and clothes.
- Staff should tie their gowns at the neck and back to cover their front and shoulders.

Be Mindful of Antimicrobial-Resistant Germs

- Identifying and treating resistant germs early helps prevent their spread.
- You can carry a resistant germ even if you do not have symptoms.
- If asked, allow health-care personnel to test you for an antimicrobial-resistant germ. Testing helps personnel choose the right antibiotic or antifungal treatment.
- Ask your provider what they and the facility will do to protect you and your family from an antimicrobial-resistant infection.

Stay Safe before and after Surgery

- Take steps, such as telling your health-care provider about other medical problems you may have and not shaving near where you will have surgery, to avoid things such as surgical site infections.[1]

[1] "Tips for Being a Safe Patient," Centers for Disease Control and Prevention (CDC), April 12, 2024. Available online. URL: www.cdc.gov/patient-safety/about/index.html. Accessed July 10, 2024.

Chapter 14 | **Medical Tourism: Benefits and Risks**

WHAT IS MEDICAL TOURISM?

Each year, millions of United States residents travel to another country for medical care, a practice known as "medical tourism." Medical tourists from the United States most commonly travel to Mexico, Canada, and several countries in Central America, South America, and the Caribbean.

REASONS FOR SEEKING MEDICAL CARE ABROAD

- **Cost**. To obtain treatment or procedures that may be cheaper in another country.
- **Culture**. To receive care from a clinician who shares the traveler's culture and language.
- **Unavailable or unapproved procedures**. To get a procedure or therapy unavailable or approved in the United States.

The most common procedures that people undergo on medical tourism trips include dental care, cosmetic surgery, fertility treatments, organ and tissue transplantation, and cancer treatment.

RISKS OF MEDICAL TOURISM

Medical tourism can be risky. The risk of complications depends on the destination, the facility where the procedure is performed, and whether the traveler is in good health for the procedure(s).

Other issues that can increase a traveler's risk of complications include:

- **Infectious diseases.** All medical procedures have some risk of infection. Complications from procedures performed in other countries include wound infections, bloodstream infections, donor-derived infections (in the case of transplantations or transfusions), and diseases such as hepatitis B, hepatitis C, and HIV.
- **Antimicrobial resistance.** Highly drug-resistant bacteria and fungi have caused disease outbreaks among medical tourists. Antimicrobial resistance happens when germs develop the ability to not respond to drugs such as antibiotics used to treat infections. Health-care facilities in other countries may not have adequate infection control practices, putting medical tourists at risk for drug-resistant infections.
- **Quality of care.** Some countries' requirements for maintaining licensure, credentialing, and accreditation may be less stringent than those in the United States. In some countries, counterfeit medicines and lower-quality medical devices may be used.
- **Communication challenges.** Communicating with staff at the destination and health-care facility may be challenging. Receiving care at a facility where you do not speak the language fluently could lead to misunderstandings about your care.
- **Air travel.** Flying after surgery can increase the risk of blood clots, including deep vein thrombosis (DVT). Delaying air travel for 10–14 days following major surgeries, particularly those involving the chest, will minimize risks associated with changes in atmospheric pressure.
- **Continuity of care.** Travelers who develop complications after returning may need to get health care in the United States. Follow-up care for complications might be expensive and prolonged and might not be covered by health insurance.

MINIMIZING MEDICAL TOURISM RISKS

Research the Clinician and Facility

- Check the qualifications of the clinician performing the procedure and the facility's credentials. Accrediting groups such as Joint Commission International (JCI), DNV GL® International Accreditation for Hospitals, and the International Society for Quality in Healthcare (ISQua) have standards for health-care facilities to meet for accreditation.
- Determine how you will communicate with your clinician and others if you do not speak the language of the destination country.

Before You Travel

- Have a pretravel consultation with your health-care provider or a travel medicine clinician at least four to six weeks before the trip to discuss healthy travel practices and specific risks.
- Obtain international travel health insurance that covers medical evacuation back to the United States.
- Find out what activities, such as swimming or hiking, are not recommended around the time of the medical procedure and plan accordingly.

Maintain Your Health and Medical Records

- Bring copies of your medical records, including lab results and other tests related to your condition and care. Inform the medical staff of any allergies.
- Pack a travel health kit with prescription and over-the-counter (OTC) medicines in their original packaging. Bring enough medicine for the entire trip, plus extra in case of delays. Also, bring copies of all prescriptions and a list of medications, including brand names, generic names, manufacturers, and dosages.
- Before returning home, get copies of all medical records from the medical facility at your destination. These may need to be translated into English.

Arrange for Follow-Up Care

- Identify where you will stay immediately after the procedure.
- Ensure you can get necessary follow-up care in the United States. Follow-up care for medical complications can be expensive and not covered by health insurance. Review health insurance policies to determine coverage and plan for the possibility of paying for additional care out-of-pocket.
- Consider supplemental travel health insurance to cover follow-up or emergency care from procedures received abroad.[1]

[1] "Medical Tourism: Travel to Another Country for Medical Care," Centers for Disease Control and Prevention (CDC), June 1, 2023. Available online. URL: wwwnc.cdc.gov/travel/page/medical-tourism. Accessed April 9, 2024.

Part 3 | Common Surgeries and Procedures

Chapter 15 | **Head and Neck Surgeries**

Chapter Contents

Section 15.1 | Treating Head and Neck Cancers

WHAT ARE CANCERS OF THE HEAD AND NECK?

Head and neck cancers usually begin in the squamous cells lining the mucosal surfaces of the head and neck, such as inside the mouth, throat, and voice box. These cancers are called "squamous cell carcinomas" (SCCs) of the head and neck. Less commonly, head and neck cancers can also begin in the salivary glands, sinuses, or muscles or nerves in the head and neck.

Areas Affected by Head and Neck Cancers

- **Oral cavity**. Includes the lips, the front two-thirds of the tongue, the gums, the lining inside the cheeks and lips, the floor of the mouth under the tongue, the hard palate, and the small area of the gum behind the wisdom teeth.
- **Throat (pharynx)**. The pharynx is a hollow tube about five inches long that starts behind the nose and leads to the esophagus. It has three parts: the nasopharynx (upper part behind the nose), the oropharynx (middle part including the soft palate, base of the tongue, and tonsils), and the hypopharynx (lower part).
- **Voice box (larynx)**. The larynx is a short passageway formed by cartilage just below the pharynx in the neck and contains the vocal cords. The epiglottis, a small piece of tissue, covers the voice box to prevent food from entering the air passages.
- **Paranasal sinuses and nasal cavity**. These are small hollow spaces in the bones of the head surrounding the nose. The nasal cavity is the hollow space inside the nose.
- **Salivary glands**. The major salivary glands are on the floor of the mouth and near the jawbone. Minor salivary glands are located throughout the mucous membranes of the mouth and throat.

Cancers of the brain, eye, esophagus, thyroid gland, and skin of the head and neck are not usually classified as head and neck cancers.

Spread and Metastasis

If an SCC of the head and neck spreads, it almost always does so locally and/or to the lymph nodes in the neck. Sometimes, cancerous squamous cells can be found in the lymph nodes of the upper neck without evidence of cancer in other parts of the head and neck, possibly due to the original primary tumor being too small. This is called "metastatic squamous cell carcinoma" with unknown (occult) primary.

TREATMENT OF HEAD AND NECK CANCERS

Treatment Options

Head and neck cancer treatment can include surgery, radiation therapy, chemotherapy, targeted therapy, immunotherapy, or a combination of treatments. The treatment plan depends on factors such as the tumor's location, the cancer stage, and the patient's age and general health.

Patients with human papillomavirus (HPV)-positive oropharyngeal tumors have a better prognosis and higher chance of complete cure than those with HPV-negative tumors following the same treatment. Clinical trials are investigating whether patients with HPV-positive cancers can be treated with less intensive regimens, such as reduced radiation or immunotherapy.

Side Effects of Treatment

- **Surgery**. It may affect the patient's ability to chew, swallow, or talk. The patient may look different after surgery, and the face and neck may be swollen, though this usually improves with time. Removal of lymph nodes can cause lymphedema, leading to additional swelling.
- **Radiation therapy**. It can cause side effects, including redness, irritation, sores in the mouth, dry mouth or thickened saliva, difficulty swallowing, changes in taste, nausea, loss of taste, earaches, and changes in skin texture. Long-term side effects include difficulty swallowing, speech impairment, and skin changes.

Patients should report any side effects to their doctor or nurse and discuss how to manage them.

REHABILITATION AND SUPPORT OPTIONS

Rehabilitation Goals

Rehabilitation aims to preserve the function of affected areas and help the patient return to normal activities as soon as possible after treatment. Rehabilitation may include physical therapy, dietary counseling, speech therapy, and learning to care for a stoma.

Reconstructive and Plastic Surgery

Patients with oral cavity cancer may need reconstructive and plastic surgery to rebuild bones or tissues. If reconstructive surgery is impossible, a prosthodontist may provide a prosthesis to restore swallowing, speech, and appearance. Patients will receive training on using the device.

Speech and Eating

Speech therapy is often necessary, and a speech-language pathologist (SLP) will plan therapy and teach exercises or alternative speaking methods. Eating may be difficult after treatment, and some patients may need a feeding tube until they can eat independently.

FOLLOW-UP CARE

Regular follow-up care is essential to ensure the cancer has not returned and a new cancer has not developed. This may include exams of the stoma, mouth, neck, and throat, regular dental exams, physical exams, blood tests, and imaging scans. If radiation is used, the doctor may monitor thyroid and pituitary gland function.

Patients are advised to stop smoking, as continued smoking can reduce treatment effectiveness and increase the risk of a second primary cancer.[1]

---

[1] "Head and Neck Cancers," National Cancer Institute (NCI), May 25, 2021. Available online. URL: www.cancer.gov/types/head-and-neck/head-neck-fact-sheet. Accessed April 18, 2024.

Section 15.2 | Brain and Spinal Cord Tumor Surgery

WHAT ARE TUMORS?

A tumor is a mass of abnormal cells forming into a new growth or was present at birth (congenital). Tumors occur when something goes wrong with genes that regulate cell growth, allowing cells to grow and divide uncontrollably. Tumors can form anywhere in the body, including the brain and spinal cord, which comprise the central nervous system (CNS).

TREATING SPINAL CORD TUMORS

A specialized team of doctors advises and assists individuals throughout treatment and rehabilitation. This team may include:

- **Neuro-oncologist**. A neurologist or oncologist specializing in CNS tumors.
- **Oncologist**. A doctor specializing in cancer.
- **Neurologist**. A doctor specializing in CNS disorders.
- **Neuroradiologist**. A doctor specializing in the CNS and trained in reading diagnostic imaging results.
- **Pathologist**. A clinical doctor who diagnoses diseases of tissues or cells using various laboratory tests.
- **Neurosurgeon**. A brain or spinal cord surgeon with specialized training in removing CNS tumors.
- **Radiation oncologist**. A doctor specializing in using radiation to treat cancer.

TREATMENT PLANS

Your health-care team will recommend a treatment plan based on the tumor's location, type, size, aggressiveness, medical history, age, and general health. Malignant tumors require treatment, while some small benign tumors may need only monitoring. Treatment for a brain or spinal tumor can include surgery, radiation therapy, chemotherapy, targeted therapy, or a combination of treatments.

Initial Treatment

Initial treatment for a CNS tumor may involve various drugs to treat or ease symptoms, including:

- anticonvulsants to treat or prevent seizures
- pain medications
- steroids or other anti-inflammatory drugs to reduce swelling and improve blood flow
- antidepressants to treat anxiety or depression following a tumor diagnosis
- antinausea drugs

Neurosurgery

Surgery is usually the first treatment to obtain tissue for diagnosis and remove as much of the tumor as possible. Surgery may be the only treatment needed if the tumor is benign or low grade. For malignant CNS tumors, surgery is best performed by a neurosurgeon.

An inaccessible or inoperable tumor cannot be removed surgically due to the risk of severe nervous system damage. These tumors are often located deep within the brain or near vital structures and may not have well-defined edges. In such cases, a biopsy may be performed to diagnose and help determine treatment.

A surgeon may insert a shunt into the skull to drain any dangerous buildup of cerebrospinal fluid (CSF) caused by the tumor. A shunt diverts the flow of CSF from the CNS to another part of the body, where it can be absorbed as part of the normal circulatory process.

SURGICAL TOOLS AND TECHNIQUES

- **Intraoperative MRI**. Provides real-time monitoring and evaluation of the surgery.
- **Navigation equipment**. Used in computer-guided neurosurgery to provide a precise, three-dimensional (3D) map of the spine or brain.
- **Intraoperative nerve monitoring**. Uses real-time recordings of nerve cell activity to monitor brain activity during surgery.

- **Surgical microscope and endoscope.** Allow surgery to be performed through a small incision in the brain or spine.

Radiation Therapy

Radiation therapy involves repeated doses of high-energy beams, such as x-rays or protons, to kill cancer cells or keep them from multiplying. It can treat surgically inaccessible tumors or tumor cells that remain following surgery.

TYPES OF RADIATION THERAPY

- **Whole brain radiation.** Shrinks multiple cancerous tumors.
- **Conventional external beam radiation.** Aims a uniform dose of high-energy radiation at the tumor and surrounding tissue.
- **Three-dimensional conformal radiotherapy (3D-CRT).** Uses diagnostic imaging to prepare an accurate, computer-generated 3D image of the tumor and surrounding tissue.
- **Intensity-modulated radiation therapy (IMRT).** Varies the intensity of radiation beams to deliver precise doses to the tumor.
- **Hyperfractionation.** Involves giving smaller amounts of radiation multiple times a day.
- **Proton beam therapy.** Directs high-energy protons at the tumor site without spreading radiation beyond the target.
- **Radiosurgery.** A one-time treatment using multiple, sharply focused radiation beams aimed at the tumor.

Side effects of radiation therapy can include fatigue, nausea, vomiting, sore skin, headache, hearing loss, sleep problems, and hair loss. Long-term effects may include shrinkage (atrophy) of the treated brain or spinal cord region.

Chemotherapy

Chemotherapy uses powerful drugs to kill cancer cells or stop them from growing or spreading. These drugs are usually given orally, intravenously, or through a catheter or port. Treatment plans depend on the type of cancer, the drugs used, and the number of cycles needed. Chemotherapy can be used before surgery (neoadjuvant therapy) or after surgery (adjuvant therapy).

Common CNS chemotherapies include temozolomide, carmustine (BCNU), lomustine (CCNU), and bevacizumab. Side effects may include hair loss, nausea, digestive problems, reduced bone marrow production, and fatigue.

Targeted Therapy

Targeted therapy uses drugs to target specific genes and proteins involved in tumor cell growth, helping to slow uncontrolled growth and reduce tumor cell production. Targeted therapies include oncogenes, growth factors, and molecules aimed at blocking gene activity.[1]

Section 15.3 | Tonsillectomy and Adenoidectomy

TONSILS

What Are Tonsils?

Tonsils are lumps of tissue at the back of the throat, with one on each side. Along with the adenoids, they are part of the lymphatic system, which clears away infection and keeps body fluids in balance. Tonsils and adenoids work by trapping germs that enter through the mouth and nose.

What Is Tonsillitis?

Tonsillitis is an inflammation (swelling) of the tonsils. Sometimes, the adenoids also swell along with the tonsils.

[1] "Brain and Spinal Cord Tumors," National Institute of Neurological Disorders and Stroke (NINDS), November 28, 2023. Available online. URL: www.ninds.nih.gov/health-information/disorders/brain-and-spinal-cord-tumors. Accessed April 18, 2024.

Causes and Risks of Tonsillitis

- **Causes.** The primary cause of tonsillitis is usually a viral infection. Bacterial infections, such as strep throat, can also cause tonsillitis.
- **Risk factors.** Tonsillitis is most common in children over age two. Almost every child in the United States gets it at least once. Bacterial tonsillitis is more common in children aged 5–15, while viral tonsillitis is more common in younger children. Adults can get tonsillitis, but it is not very common.

Is Tonsillitis Contagious?

Although tonsillitis is not contagious, the viruses and bacteria that cause it are contagious. Frequent handwashing can help prevent the spread of infections.

Symptoms of Tonsillitis

- severe sore throat
- red, swollen tonsils
- trouble swallowing
- white or yellow coating on the tonsils
- swollen glands in the neck
- fever
- bad breath

When to See a Health-Care Provider

Call your health-care provider if your child:

- has a sore throat for more than two days
- has trouble or pain when swallowing
- feels very sick or very weak

Seek emergency care if your child:

- has trouble breathing
- starts drooling
- has a lot of trouble swallowing

Diagnosing Tonsillitis

To diagnose tonsillitis, the health-care provider will examine your child's throat and neck and may perform one or more tests for strep throat. These tests include a rapid strep test and a throat culture.

Treatments for Tonsillitis

Treatment depends on the cause:

- **Viral tonsillitis.** No specific medicine is available.
- **Bacterial tonsillitis.** Antibiotics are prescribed. It is crucial to complete the full course of antibiotics.

TIPS FOR COMFORT

- Ensure your child gets plenty of rest.
- Encourage fluid intake.
- Provide soft foods if swallowing is painful.
- Offer warm liquids or cold foods such as Popsicles.
- Avoid exposure to cigarette smoke or other irritants.
- Use a humidifier in the child's room.
- Encourage gargling with salt water.
- Offer lozenges (not for children under age four).
- Use over-the-counter (OTC) pain relievers like acetaminophen (avoid aspirin for children and teenagers).

What Is a Tonsillectomy?

A tonsillectomy is surgery to remove the tonsils. It may be necessary if your child:

- frequently gets tonsillitis
- has bacterial tonsillitis that does not respond to antibiotics
- has enlarged tonsils, causing trouble breathing or swallowing

Most children go home the same day, but very young children or those with complications may need to stay overnight. Recovery typically takes one to two weeks.[1]

---

[1] MedlinePlus, "Tonsillitis," National Institutes of Health (NIH), April 11, 2017. Available online. URL: https://medlineplus.gov/tonsillitis.html. Accessed April 8, 2024.

ADENOIDS

What Are Adenoids?

Adenoids are a patch of tissue high in the throat, just behind the nose. They are part of the lymphatic system and work alongside the tonsils to trap germs. Adenoids usually start to shrink after about age five and are almost completely gone by the teenage years.

Enlarged Adenoids

CAUSES

- **Congenital.** Some children are born with enlarged adenoids.
- **Infections.** Adenoids can become enlarged when fighting infections and might remain swollen afterward.

SYMPTOMS

- difficulty breathing through the nose
- mouth breathing
- dry mouth and bad breath
- cracked lips
- runny nose
- loud breathing
- snoring
- restless sleep
- sleep apnea
- ear infections

DIAGNOSIS

Health-care providers diagnose enlarged adenoids by:

- reviewing medical history and symptoms
- examining the ears, throat, and mouth
- feeling the neck

To check the size of the adenoids, providers may use a special mirror, an endoscope, or an x-ray.

Treatments for Enlarged Adenoids

Treatment depends on the severity of symptoms:

- **Mild symptoms**. May not require treatment.
- **Medications**. Nasal sprays or antibiotics for bacterial infections.
- **Adenoidectomy**. Surgery to remove the adenoids if there are repeated infections, antibiotic-resistant infections, or blocked airways.

What Is an Adenoidectomy?

An adenoidectomy is surgery to remove the adenoids. It is recommended for children with repeated adenoid infections, resistant bacterial infections, or enlarged adenoids that block airways. If there is also a problem with the tonsils, a tonsillectomy may be performed simultaneously. Most children go home the same day, but recovery can take several days.[2]

Section 15.4 | Tympanostomy Tubes in Pediatric Otitis Media

Uncertainty about the comparative effectiveness of tympanostomy tubes for children with otitis media (OM), indications for tympanostomy in children, antibiotic prescriptions for children with tube otorrhea, and prophylactic water precaution devices prompted the Agency for Healthcare Research and Quality (AHRQ) to commission a review. This review will inform recommendations concerning surgical indications and management strategies for tympanostomy tube placement.

PATHOGENESIS OF OTITIS MEDIA

Otitis media often begins with a viral upper respiratory tract infection that causes Eustachian tube obstruction, negative

[2] MedlinePlus, "Adenoids," National Institutes of Health (NIH), September 13, 2022. Available online. URL: https://medlineplus.gov/adenoids.html. Accessed April 8, 2024.

middle ear pressure, and fluid accumulation in this normally air-filled space.

- **Acute otitis media (AOM).** Defined as fluid in the middle ear with signs and symptoms of an acute infection, such as fever and ear pain.
- **Otitis media with effusion (OME).** Defined as fluid in the middle ear behind an intact tympanic membrane without signs and symptoms of an acute infection. It is considered chronic OME if effusion persists for three months or longer.

Children with chronic OME are prone to recurrent AOM episodes. After an AOM episode, all children have OME for some time. Myringotomy with tympanostomy tube placement is the most common ambulatory surgery performed on children in the United States, with almost 700,000 procedures yearly at an estimated annual cost of $1.8 billion.

INDICATIONS FOR TYMPANOSTOMY TUBE PLACEMENT

In 1994, indications for tympanostomy tube placement in children were reported as follows:

- 30 percent for persistent OME
- 24 percent for recurrent AOM
- 46 percent for both recurrent AOM and persistent OME

RISKS AND BENEFITS OF TYMPANOSTOMY TUBES

Chronic OME can result in hearing deficits, potentially leading to speech and language delays, behavioral changes, and poor academic achievement. Recurrent AOM can affect the quality of life (QOL) for patients and caregivers. The comparative effectiveness of tympanostomy tubes for chronic OME and recurrent AOM is influenced by factors such as the child's age, age at first diagnosis, frequency of respiratory tract infections, and daycare exposure.

Children with bilateral and continuous middle ear effusions are at higher risk. A risk-centered approach should incorporate important determinants of outcome rather than a single threshold for the duration or frequency of diagnosis.

Certain children, including those with Down syndrome and cleft palate, are at very high risk for middle ear disease and may require multiple sets of tubes during childhood. Children with autism spectrum disorder also have a higher likelihood of undergoing tympanostomy tube placement.

RECOMMENDATIONS BY PROFESSIONAL ORGANIZATIONS

The American Academy of Otolaryngology-Head and Neck Surgery (AAO-HNS) clinical practice guideline (CPG) recommends that clinicians offer tympanostomy tubes to children with recurrent AOM and middle ear effusions based on shared decision-making with the child's caregiver. They conclude that tubes should not be placed in children with recurrent AOM who have a normal ear examination at the time of assessment for tube candidacy. The American Academy of Pediatrics (AAP) CPG discourages routine use of prophylactic antibiotics to prevent recurrent AOM due to concerns about antibiotic resistance.

WATER PRECAUTIONS AND POSTOPERATIVE CARE

A 2014 review by Gabriel J. Tsao, ENT-otolaryngologist in Point Richmond and Richard L. Goode, MD, otolaryngologist at the Stanford University School of Medicine, concluded that water precautions should not be routinely advised to prevent post-tympanostomy tube otorrhea. Acute otorrhea is common after tympanostomy tube placement, reflecting underlying middle ear changes and inflammation. Treatment aims to eradicate bacterial infection using antibiotic eardrops with or without glucocorticoids.

OBJECTIVES OF THE SYSTEMATIC REVIEW

The objectives for the systematic review are to evaluate:

- the effectiveness of tympanostomy tubes in children with chronic OM with effusion and recurrent AOM
- the frequency of adverse effects and/or complications associated with tympanostomy tube placement

- the necessity for water precautions in children with tympanostomy tubes
- the comparative effectiveness of available treatments for otorrhea in children with this complication

This review by AHRQ aims to provide comprehensive evidence to guide clinical decision-making regarding tympanostomy tube placement in children with OM. The review will help clinicians and caregivers make informed decisions about managing this common condition in pediatric patients.[1]

Section 15.5 | **Cochlear Implants**

WHAT IS A COCHLEAR IMPLANT?

A cochlear implant is a small, complex electronic device that provides a sense of sound to individuals who are profoundly deaf or severely hard-of-hearing. The implant consists of an external portion that sits behind the ear and a second portion that is surgically placed under the skin (see Figure 15.1). An implant has the following parts:

- **Microphone**. It picks up sound from the environment.
- **Speech processor**. It selects and arranges sounds picked up by the microphone.
- **Transmitter and receiver/stimulator**. It receives signals from the speech processor and converts them into electric impulses.
- **Electrode array**. It collects the impulses from the stimulator and sends them to different regions of the auditory nerve.

A cochlear implant does not restore normal hearing but provides a useful representation of sounds to help understand speech.

[1] Agency for Healthcare Research and Quality (AHRQ), "Tympanostomy Tubes," U.S. Department of Health and Human Services (HHS), March 2021. Available online. URL: https://effectivehealthcare.ahrq.gov/products/tympanostomy-tubes/research-protocol. Accessed July 10, 2024.

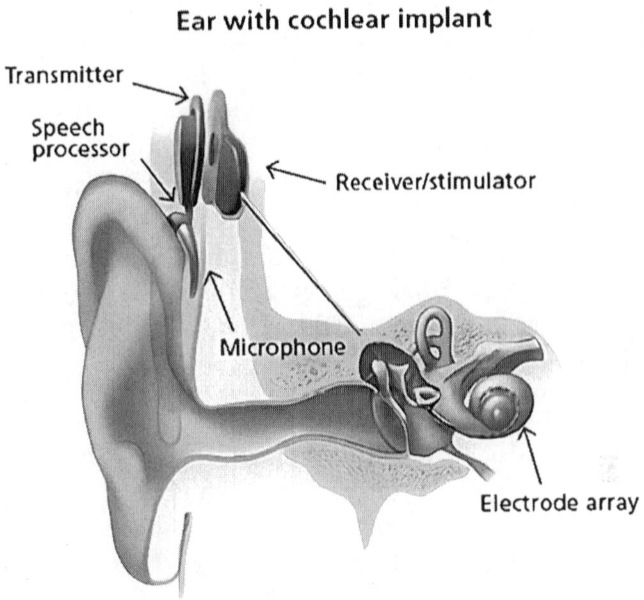

Figure 15.1. Ear with Cochlear Implant

National Institute on Deafness and Other Communication Disorders (NIDCD)

HOW DOES A COCHLEAR IMPLANT WORK?

A cochlear implant is different from a hearing aid. While hearing aids amplify sounds to be detected by damaged ears, cochlear implants bypass damaged portions of the ear and directly stimulate the auditory nerve. Signals generated by the implant are sent to the brain via the auditory nerve, which recognizes these signals as sound. Hearing through a cochlear implant differs from normal hearing and requires time to learn or relearn. However, it enables many people to recognize warning signals, understand environmental sounds, and comprehend speech in person or over the telephone.

RECEIVING A COCHLEAR IMPLANT

The process involves both a surgical procedure and significant therapy to learn or relearn the sense of hearing. Not everyone performs at the same level with this device. The decision to receive an implant should involve discussions with medical specialists, including an experienced cochlear-implant surgeon. The process can be expensive, and while some health insurance plans may cover the cost, not all do. Individuals may choose not to have a cochlear implant for various personal reasons. Surgical implantation is generally safe, although complications are a risk factor, as with any surgery. Learning to interpret the sounds created by an implant requires time and practice, often involving speech-language pathologists (SLPs) and audiologists. These factors should be considered before implantation.[1]

PRE-SURGERY PROCEDURES

Patients are usually referred by primary care doctors to ear, nose, and throat (ENT) doctors for evaluation. Common tests include:

- examination of the external, middle, and inner ear for signs of infection or abnormality
- various hearing tests, such as an audiogram
- a trial of hearing aid use to assess potential benefit
- exams to evaluate middle and inner ear structures:
    - **Computed tomography (CT) scan**. It helps determine if the cochlea has a normal shape, which is especially important for patients with a history of meningitis.
    - **Magnetic resonance imaging (MRI) scan**. It provides detailed images of ear structures.
- psychological examination to assess if the patient can cope with the implant
- physical exam to prepare for general anesthesia

DURING SURGERY

The surgical procedure involves:

- inserting intravenous (IV) lines

[1] "Cochlear Implants," National Institute on Deafness and Other Communication Disorders (NIDCD), April 1, 2024. Available online. URL: www.nidcd.nih.gov/health/cochlear-implants. Accessed April 18, 2024.

- shaving or cleaning the scalp around the implant site
- attaching cables, monitors, and patches to monitor vital signs
- providing oxygen and anesthetic gas through a mask
- administering drugs to induce sleep and general anesthesia
- awakening the patient in the operating room and transferring them to a recovery room until the anesthesia wears off

POST-SURGERY CARE

Immediately after waking, a patient may experience:

- pressure or discomfort over the implanted ear
- dizziness
- nausea
- disorientation or confusion
- sore throat from the breathing tube used during anesthesia

Subsequently, the patient can expect to:

- keep bandages on for a while, which may be stained with blood or fluid
- go home about a day after surgery
- have stitches for a while and receive instructions on caring for them
- have an appointment in about a week to remove stitches and examine the implant site
- have the implant turned on (activated) about three to six weeks later

ACTIVATION AND FOLLOW-UP

Without the external transmitter, the patient cannot hear. The clinic provides the external components about a month after surgery during the first programming session. This waiting period allows the operative incision to heal completely. After the swelling subsides, an audiologist adjusts the sound processor to fit the implanted patient, tests to ensure correct adjustments, determines what sounds the patient hears, and provides information on proper care and use of the device.[2]

[2] "Before, during, and after Implant Surgery," U.S. Food and Drug Administration (FDA), December 29, 2017. Available online. URL: www.fda.gov/medical-devices/cochlear-implants/during-after-implant-surgery. Accessed April 18, 2024.

Chapter 16 | Eye Surgeries

Chapter Contents

Section 16.1 | Cataract Surgery

WHAT IS A CATARACT?

A cataract is a cloudy area in the lens of your eye, which is the clear part that helps to focus light. This condition can make your vision cloudy. Surgery is the only way to remove cataracts.

WHO NEEDS CATARACT SURGERY?

Your eye doctor may suggest cataract surgery if your vision loss interferes with everyday activities such as reading, driving, or watching TV. Surgery might also be recommended even if cataracts are not the main cause of your vision problems, such as when the doctor needs to see into the back of your eye to track and treat other conditions such as diabetic retinopathy (DR) or age-related macular degeneration (AMD).

You do not need to rush into surgery. Discuss the risks and benefits with your eye doctor to decide if surgery is right for you. If you have cataracts in both eyes, surgery will be done on each eye separately, usually about a month apart.

HOW TO PREPARE FOR CATARACT SURGERY

Your eye doctor will provide specific instructions to prepare for your cataract surgery. General steps include:

- **Visit your eye doctor**. About a week before surgery, your eye doctor will perform tests to measure the size and shape of your eye to select the right kind of artificial lens (intraocular lens or IOL).
- **Use special eye drops**. Prescribed eye drops help protect your eye from infection.
- **Stop taking certain medications**. Inform your doctor about any medications you take. You may need to stop taking medications that could cause bleeding during surgery.
- **Fasting**. Do not eat or drink for several hours before surgery.

- **Clean your eyelids and eyelashes.** Use baby shampoo to clean your eyelids and eyelashes the night before and the morning of surgery to remove any germs that could cause infection.

THE DAY OF YOUR SURGERY

Bring a friend or family member, as you will not be able to drive after the surgery. They can help ensure you get home safely.

WHAT HAPPENS DURING CATARACT SURGERY?

During the approximately one-hour procedure, your eye doctor will:

- administer numbing drops to your eye
- use tiny tools to cut into your eye, break up the cloudy lens, and remove it
- place the new artificial lens (IOL) in your eye

You will be awake but will not feel or see the procedure. After the surgery, you will rest in a recovery area until the anesthesia wears off. The medical team will check for any immediate problems before you go home.

POST-SURGERY CARE

After surgery, your eye doctor will provide instructions on how to protect your eye, including:

- using prescribed eye drops to aid in healing
- wearing a special eye shield or glasses
- avoiding certain activities like touching your eye, bending over, or lifting heavy objects for a few weeks

Your eye may feel itchy, uncomfortable, and sensitive to light and touch initially. These symptoms should improve within a day or two.

Call your eye doctor immediately if you experience vision loss, severe pain, very red eyes, or see floaters (flashes of light or dark spots).

VISION AFTER CATARACT SURGERY

Most people see better after cataract surgery, although vision may initially be blurry. Colors may appear brighter because the artificial lens does not have the yellow or brown tint of the cataract. You may need a new prescription for glasses or contact lenses once your eye has completely healed.

RISKS OF CATARACT SURGERY

Cataract surgery is common, safe, and effective, but risks include:

- swelling, bleeding, or infections
- vision loss or double vision
- unusual changes in eye pressure
- retinal detachment
- secondary cataracts or posterior capsule opacity (PCO)

Your eye doctor can treat these issues, but early treatment is crucial. Attend all follow-up appointments and contact your doctor if you notice any problems with your eyes or vision.[1]

Section 16.2 | Understanding Glaucoma and Its Surgical Treatments

WHAT IS GLAUCOMA?

Glaucoma is a group of eye diseases that can cause vision loss and blindness by damaging the optic nerve, located at the back of the eye.

If glaucoma medications and laser treatments have not been effective, your doctor may recommend surgery. While surgery cannot cure glaucoma or reverse vision loss, it can help protect your vision and prevent it from worsening.

[1] "Cataract Surgery," National Eye Institute (NEI), January 4, 2023. Available online. URL: www.nei.nih.gov/learn-about-eye-health/eye-conditions-and-diseases/cataracts/cataract-surgery. Accessed April 18, 2024.

WHAT ARE THE TYPES OF GLAUCOMA SURGERY?

Several types of glaucoma surgery can help lower eye pressure, including:

- trabeculectomy
- glaucoma implant surgery
- minimally invasive glaucoma surgery (MIGS)

If surgery is needed for both eyes, the procedures will be performed on one eye at a time.

What Is Trabeculectomy?

This type of surgery is typically used to treat open-angle glaucoma. It is performed in a hospital and usually takes less than an hour.

During the procedure, the surgeon creates a tiny opening in the top of the eye, beneath the eyelid, where it is not visible. This opening allows excess fluid to drain away, reducing eye pressure.

You will usually be awake during the surgery but will receive numbing medication and medication to help you relax. Most patients can go home the same day, but you will need someone to drive you home.

What Is Glaucoma Implant Surgery?

This surgery treats various types of glaucoma, including congenital glaucoma, neovascular glaucoma, and glaucoma caused by an injury. It is performed in a hospital and typically takes one to two hours.

In this procedure, the surgeon implants a tiny tube, or shunt, onto the white part of the eye. The tube helps drain excess fluid, lowering eye pressure.

You will be awake during the surgery but will receive numbing medication and medication to help you relax. Most patients can go home the same day, but you will need someone to drive you home.

What Is Minimally Invasive Glaucoma Surgery?

For mild glaucoma, your doctor may recommend a new approach called "MIGS." This method also lowers eye pressure but has fewer risks and side effects, allowing faster recovery.

There are different types of MIGS, so consult your eye doctor to determine if this option suits you.

WHAT HAPPENS AFTER SURGERY?

Your doctor will prescribe eye drops to help prevent swelling and infections. These drops differ from other glaucoma drops you may already use and must be used for several weeks.

During recovery, you may need to avoid certain activities, such as lifting heavy objects, for two to four weeks. Regular checkups with your doctor are necessary to ensure proper healing.

WILL YOU NEED SURGERY AGAIN?

The benefits of surgery can vary. Some people experience long-term relief, while others may require additional surgery if the opening in the eye starts to close. Regular eye pressure checkups are essential to monitor and address any issues promptly.

Research indicates that trabeculectomy can lower eye pressure in about 7 out of 10 people, with the best results seen in those without a history of eye injury or surgery.

WHAT ARE THE SIDE EFFECTS OF GLAUCOMA SURGERY?

Like any surgery, glaucoma surgery can have side effects. These may include:

- eye swelling and soreness
- cataract
- corneal problems
- low eye pressure
- vision loss

Discuss the pros and cons of surgery with your doctor to create a treatment plan that suits your needs.[1]

[1] "Glaucoma Surgery," National Eye Institute (NEI), January 3, 2022. Available online. URL: www.nei.nih.gov/learn-about-eye-health/eye-conditions-and-diseases/glaucoma/glaucoma-surgery. Accessed April 18, 2024.

Section 16.3 | Phakic Intraocular Lens Implantation Surgery

WHAT ARE PHAKIC INTRAOCULAR LENSES?

Phakic intraocular lenses, or phakic lenses, are plastic or silicone lenses implanted permanently into the eye to reduce the need for glasses or contact lenses. The term "phakic" refers to the fact that the natural lens of the eye is left intact during the implantation. During phakic lens implantation surgery, a small incision is made in the front of the eye. The phakic lens is then inserted through the incision and placed either just in front of or just behind the iris.

WHAT DO PHAKIC INTRAOCULAR LENSES TREAT?

Phakic lenses correct refractive errors, which are imperfections in the eye's focusing power. All phakic lenses approved by the U.S. Food and Drug Administration (FDA) are designed to correct nearsightedness (myopia).

The cornea and natural lens focus light to create an image on the retina, similar to how a camera lens focuses light onto film. This process, known as "refraction," can be disrupted by refractive errors, causing blurred or out-of-focus images on the retina.

Nearsighted individuals have difficulty seeing distant objects clearly, as the images of them come into focus in front of the retina instead of on it. Phakic lenses aim to correct this by focusing light directly on the retina, providing clear distance vision without glasses or contact lenses.

ALTERNATIVES TO PHAKIC LENSES

Surgery is not the only option for correcting nearsightedness. Glasses or contact lenses can also correct vision. Other surgical options include photorefractive keratectomy (PRK) and laser-assisted in situ keratomileusis (LASIK), depending on the degree of nearsightedness and other eye conditions.

CAN PHAKIC INTRAOCULAR LENSES BE REMOVED?

Phakic lenses are intended to be permanent, although they can be surgically removed. However, returning to your previous level of vision or eye condition cannot be guaranteed after removal.

RISKS ASSOCIATED WITH PHAKIC INTRAOCULAR LENSES

Like any medical procedure, implanting a phakic lens involves risks. Understanding these risks and limitations is crucial before deciding to undergo surgery.

Potential risks include:

- **Vision loss**. Some patients may experience vision loss that cannot be corrected with glasses, contact lenses, or surgery.
- **Debilitating visual symptoms**. Glare, halos, double vision, and decreased vision in low light can occur, affecting tasks such as night driving.
- **Need for additional surgery**. Further procedures may be required to reposition, replace, or remove the phakic lens due to improper lens power or position.
- **Under- or over-treatment**. Achieving a perfect 20/20 vision is not guaranteed, and additional corrective measures may be necessary.
- **Increased intraocular pressure**. Post-surgery pressure increases may require medication or additional surgery to manage.
- **Corneal clouding**. A decrease in endothelial cells can lead to a cloudy cornea and potential vision loss, possibly necessitating a corneal transplant.
- **Cataract development**. The risk of cataracts may increase, potentially requiring cataract surgery.
- **Retinal detachment**. The risk of retinal detachment increases after intraocular surgery.
- **Infection, bleeding, or severe inflammation**. Rare but serious complications can lead to permanent vision loss or loss of the eye.

- **Unknown long-term risks**. Phakic lenses are a relatively new technology, and long-term risks are not fully known.

BEFORE SURGERY

Initial Visit

Before deciding on phakic intraocular lens implantation, you will undergo an initial examination to ensure your eye is healthy and suitable for surgery. This examination includes a complete medical and eye health history and thorough eye measurements.

If you wear contact lenses, your doctor may ask you to stop wearing them before the examination to ensure accurate measurements.

Deciding to Have Surgery

Discuss with your doctor whether you are a good candidate for phakic lenses and understand the risks, benefits, and alternatives. Ask questions and review any provided informational literature. Do not feel pressured to decide, and carefully consider all aspects before signing an informed consent document.

Preparing for Surgery

You may undergo a laser iridotomy to prepare your eye about one to two weeks before surgery. This procedure, performed in an office or clinic, involves making a small hole in the iris to prevent fluid buildup and pressure.

Your doctor may also ask you to stop taking certain medications before surgery to reduce the risk of bleeding. You will receive prescriptions for antibiotics and anti-inflammatory drops to use before and after surgery.

DURING SURGERY

On the day of surgery, numbing drops will be administered, and you will need to lie still. Sedatives or other medications may be given to help you relax. The surgeon will make an incision, insert the phakic lens, and use stitches to close the incision. The surgery usually takes about 30 minutes.

AFTER SURGERY

Immediate Post-Surgery

You may experience light sensitivity and minor discomfort. Follow your doctor's instructions for using prescribed drops and wearing an eye shield. Your vision may be hazy or blurry initially but should improve over time.

Long-Term Care

Regular follow-up visits are crucial to monitor your progress and manage any complications. Annual eye exams are recommended, and you should maintain records of endothelial cell counts. Notify your eye doctor of any vision changes or issues, and protect your eyes during activities that could cause injury.

By following these guidelines and understanding the risks and benefits, you can make an informed decision about phakic intraocular lens implantation surgery.[1]

Section 16.4 | **Understanding LASIK Surgery**

Laser-assisted in situ keratomileusis (LASIK) is a procedure that permanently changes the shape of the cornea, the clear covering of the front of the eye, using an excimer laser. A mechanical microkeratome (a blade device) or a laser keratome (a laser device) is used to cut a flap in the cornea. A hinge is left at one end of this flap. The flap is folded back, revealing the stroma, the middle section of the cornea. Pulses from a computer-controlled laser vaporize a portion of the stroma, and then the flap is replaced.

RISKS AND FINDING THE RIGHT DOCTOR

Most patients are pleased with the results of their refractive surgery. However, like any medical procedure, there are risks involved.

[1] "Phakic Intraocular Lenses," U.S. Food and Drug Administration (FDA), March 26, 2018. Available online. URL: www.fda.gov/medical-devices/implants-and-prosthetics/phakic-intraocular-lenses. Accessed April 18, 2024.

Understanding these risks and limitations is crucial before deciding to undergo surgery.

Potential risks include:

- **Vision loss.** Some patients lose lines of vision on the vision chart that cannot be corrected with glasses, contact lenses, or surgery due to treatment.
- **Debilitating visual symptoms.** Some patients develop glare, halos, and/or double vision, which can seriously affect nighttime vision. Even with good vision on the vision chart, some patients do not see as well in low-contrast situations, such as at night or in fog.
- **Under- or over-treatment.** Only a certain percentage of patients achieve 20/20 vision without glasses or contacts. Additional treatment may be required, but it may not be possible. Glasses or contact lenses might still be needed post-surgery.
- **Severe dry eye syndrome.** The eye may not produce enough tears to remain moist and comfortable, causing discomfort and reduced visual quality. This condition may be permanent, requiring intensive drop therapy and the use of plugs or other procedures.
- **Large refractive errors.** Results are generally not as good in patients with very large refractive errors. You should discuss your expectations with your doctor and realize that you may still require glasses or contacts after the surgery.
- **Farsighted patients.** For some farsighted patients, the results may diminish with age. The level of improved vision experienced after surgery may decrease over time.
- **Long-term data.** LASIK is a relatively new technology, with the first laser approved for LASIK eye surgery in 1998. Therefore, the long-term safety and effectiveness of LASIK surgery are not fully known.

PREPARING FOR LASIK SURGERY

Before Surgery

If you decide to proceed with LASIK surgery, you will need an initial or baseline evaluation by your eye doctor to determine if you are a good candidate. This is what you need to know to prepare for the exam and what to expect:

- **Contact lenses**. If you wear contact lenses, stop wearing them before your baseline evaluation and switch to wearing glasses full-time. Contact lenses can change the shape of your cornea, affecting measurements and surgical planning.
  - **Soft contact lenses**. Stop wearing them for two weeks before your initial evaluation.
  - **Toric soft lenses or rigid gas-permeable (RGP) lenses**. Stop wearing them for at least three weeks before your initial evaluation.
  - **Hard lenses**. Stop wearing them for at least four weeks before your initial evaluation.
- **Medical history**. Inform your doctor about your past and present medical and eye conditions, all medications you take, including over-the-counter (OTC) medications, and any allergies.
- **Eye exam**. Your doctor will perform a thorough eye exam and discuss:
  - whether you are a good candidate
  - the risks, benefits, and alternatives of the surgery
  - what to expect before, during, and after surgery
  - your responsibilities before, during, and after surgery
- **Decision-making**. Give yourself plenty of time to think about the risk/benefit discussion, review any informational literature provided, and have any additional questions answered by your doctor before deciding to proceed with surgery.

Preparing for Surgery

- **Day before surgery**. Stop using creams, lotions, makeup, and perfumes to reduce the risk of infection.

Your doctor may ask you to scrub your eyelashes to remove residues.

- **Transportation**. Arrange for transportation to and from your surgery and your first follow-up visit.
- **Medication**. Your doctor may give you medicine to help you relax on the day of surgery. Ensure someone can bring you home after surgery, as your vision may be blurry, and you may be impaired.

DURING SURGERY

Creating the Flap

- **Mechanical microkeratome**. If a mechanical microkeratome is used, a ring is placed on your eye, and very high pressure is applied to create suction. Your vision will dim while the suction ring is on, and you may feel the pressure and experience some discomfort during this part of the procedure. The microkeratome, a cutting instrument, is attached to the suction ring. Your doctor will use the microkeratome blade to cut a flap in your cornea. Microkeratome blades are meant to be used only once and then discarded.
  The microkeratome and the suction ring are then removed.
- **Laser keratome**. If a laser keratome is used, the cornea is flattened with a clear plastic plate. Your vision will dim, and you may feel the pressure and experience some discomfort during this part of the procedure. Laser energy is focused inside the cornea tissue, creating thousands of small bubbles of gas and water that expand and connect to separate the tissue underneath the cornea surface, creating a flap. The plate is then removed.

You can see, but you will experience fluctuating degrees of blurred vision during the rest of the procedure. The doctor will lift the flap, fold it back on its hinge, and dry the exposed tissue.

Laser Treatment

The laser will be positioned over your eye, and you will be asked to stare at a light. This is not the laser used to remove tissue from the cornea. This light helps you keep your eye fixed on one spot once the laser is activated.

When your eye is in the correct position, your doctor will start the laser. At this point in the surgery, you may become aware of new sounds and smells. The pulse of the laser makes a ticking sound. As the laser removes corneal tissue, some people report a smell similar to burning hair. A computer controls the amount of laser energy delivered to your eye. Before surgery, your doctor will have programmed the computer to vaporize a particular amount of tissue based on the measurements taken at your initial evaluation. After the pulses of laser energy vaporize the corneal tissue, the flap is put back into position.

At the end of the procedure, a shield should be placed over your eye to protect it, as no stitches are used to hold the flap in place. It is important to wear this shield to prevent you from rubbing your eye and putting pressure on your eye while you sleep and to protect your eye from being accidentally hit or poked until the flap has healed.

AFTER SURGERY

Immediate Post-Surgery

- **Discomfort**. Your eye may burn, itch, or feel like something is in it. You may experience some discomfort or mild pain, and your doctor may suggest a mild pain reliever. Both your eyes may tear or water. Your vision will probably be hazy or blurry. Avoid rubbing your eye, as this could dislodge the flap, requiring further treatment.
- **Symptoms**. You may experience sensitivity to light, glare, starbursts, or halos around lights. The whites of your eye may look red or bloodshot. These symptoms should improve within the first few days after surgery. Plan to take a few days off from work until these symptoms subside.

Follow-Up Care

You should see your doctor within 24–48 hours after surgery and at regular intervals for at least the first six months. At the first postoperative visit, your doctor will remove the eye shield, test your vision, and examine your eye. Your doctor may give you one or more types of eye drops to help prevent infection and/or inflammation. You may also be advised to use artificial tears to help lubricate the eye. Do not resume wearing a contact lens in the operated eye, even if your vision is blurry.

You should wait one to three days following surgery before beginning any noncontact sports, depending on the activity level required, how you feel, and your doctor's instructions.

To help prevent infection, you may need to wait up to two weeks after surgery before using lotions, creams, or makeup around the eye. Your doctor may advise you to continue scrubbing your eyelashes for a period of time after surgery. Avoid swimming and using hot tubs or whirlpools for one to two months.

Strenuous contact sports such as boxing, football, or karate should not be attempted for at least four weeks after surgery. It is important to protect your eyes from anything that might get into them and from being hit or bumped.

Recovery Period

During the first few months after surgery, your vision may fluctuate. It may take up to three to six months for your vision to stabilize. Glare, halos, difficulty driving at night, and other visual symptoms may persist during this stabilization period. If further correction or enhancement is necessary, you should wait until your eye measurements are consistent for two consecutive visits at least three months apart before reoperation. Although distance vision may improve after reoperation, other visual symptoms, such as glare or halos, are unlikely to improve.

LONG-TERM CARE

No laser company has presented enough evidence for the U.S. Food and Drug Administration (FDA) to make conclusions about the safety or effectiveness of enhancement surgery. Contact your eye doctor immediately if you develop any new, unusual, or worsening symptoms at any point after surgery. Such symptoms could signal a problem that, if not treated early enough, may lead to vision loss.[1]

[1] "LASIK," U.S. Food and Drug Administration (FDA), October 7, 2022. Available online. URL: www.fda.gov/medical-devices/surgery-devices/lasik. Accessed April 18, 2024.

Chapter 17 | **Dental and Oral Surgeries**

Chapter Contents

Section 17.1 | Dental Implants

When a tooth is lost due to injury or disease, complications such as rapid bone loss, defective speech, or changes in chewing patterns can arise, resulting in discomfort. Replacing a lost tooth with a dental implant can significantly enhance a person's quality of life (QOL) and overall health.

Dental implants are medical devices surgically implanted into the jaw to restore a person's ability to chew or their appearance. They provide support for artificial teeth, such as crowns, bridges, or dentures.

COMPONENTS OF DENTAL IMPLANT SYSTEMS

Dental implant systems consist of:

- **Dental implant body**. Surgically inserted in the jawbone, replacing the tooth's root.
- **Dental implant abutment**. Attached to the implant body by the abutment fixation screw, extending through the gums to support the attached artificial teeth.
- **Abutment fixation screw**. It may be included to secure the abutment to the implant body.

CONSIDERATIONS BEFORE CHOOSING DENTAL IMPLANTS

Before opting for dental implants, discuss with your dental provider the potential benefits and risks, and whether you are a suitable candidate for the procedure. Consider the following factors:

- **Overall health**. Your general health is crucial in determining your candidacy for dental implants, the healing duration, and the longevity of the implant.
- **Implant information**. Ask your dental provider about the brand and model of the dental implant system, and keep this information for your records.
- **Smoking**. Smoking can affect the healing process and decrease the long-term success of the implant.

- **Healing process.** The implant body may take several months or longer to heal, during which you typically have a temporary abutment in place of the tooth.

POST-PROCEDURE CARE

After the dental implant procedure, follow these guidelines for long-term success:

- **Oral hygiene.** Adhere to the oral hygiene instructions provided by your dental provider. Regular cleaning of the implant and surrounding teeth is essential.
- **Regular visits.** Schedule regular visits with your dental provider.
- **Implant issues.** Inform your dental provider immediately if your implant feels loose or painful.

BENEFITS AND RISKS OF DENTAL IMPLANT SYSTEMS

Benefits

- **Restores ability to chew.** Enables normal chewing function.
- **Cosmetic appearance.** Improves the visual aspect of your teeth.
- **Prevents bone loss.** Helps prevent jawbone shrinkage due to bone loss.
- **Preserves oral health.** Maintains the health of surrounding bone and gums.
- **Stabilizes adjacent teeth.** Helps keep nearby teeth stable.
- **Improves QOL.** Enhances overall well-being and confidence.

Risks

- **Damage to surrounding teeth.** It can occur during implant placement.
- **Tissue injury.** Possible injury to surrounding tissues during surgery, such as sinus perforation.
- **Jawbone fracture.** Risk of fracturing the surrounding jawbone during surgery.

- **Inadequate function.** The implant may feel unnatural or fail to bite correctly.
- **Implant looseness.** The abutment screw may loosen, causing the tooth to feel loose or twist in place.
- **Implant failure.** It can occur due to systemic infection (more likely in patients with uncontrolled diabetes), local infection in the bone and gums, or delayed healing (more likely in smokers).
- **Oral hygiene issues.** Difficulty cleaning the gums around the implant can lead to poor oral hygiene.
- **Periodontal disease.** Untreated gum disease can affect the implant.
- **Nerve damage.** Postsurgical numbness due to nerve impingement or damage.

PRECAUTIONS

Always notify health-care providers and imaging technicians about your dental implants before any magnetic resonance imaging (MRI) or x-ray procedures. Dental implants can distort or interfere with these images.[1]

Section 17.2 | Surgical Treatments for Periodontal (Gum) Disease

WHAT IS PERIODONTAL (GUM) DISEASE?

If you have been diagnosed with periodontal (gum) disease, you are not alone. Many adults in the United States have some form of this disease. Periodontal diseases range from simple gum inflammation to severe conditions that cause significant damage to the soft tissue and bone supporting the teeth. In the worst cases, teeth are lost.

[1] "Dental Implants: What You Should Know," U.S. Food and Drug Administration (FDA), October 29, 2021. Available online. URL: www.fda.gov/medical-devices/dental-devices/dental-implants-what-you-should-know. Accessed April 18, 2024.

From this point forward, the progression of gum disease greatly depends on how well you care for your teeth and gums daily.

SURGICAL TREATMENTS

Flap Surgery

Surgery may be necessary if inflammation and deep pockets persist following deep cleaning and medication treatments. A dentist or periodontist might perform flap surgery to remove tartar deposits in deep pockets or reduce the periodontal pocket, making it easier to keep the area clean. This common surgery involves lifting the gums back and removing the tartar. The gums are then sutured back so the tissue fits snugly around the tooth again. After surgery, the gums will heal and fit more tightly around the tooth, sometimes making the teeth appear longer.

Bone and Tissue Grafts

In addition to flap surgery, your periodontist or dentist may suggest procedures to help regenerate any bone or gum tissue lost due to periodontitis.

- **Bone grafting**. Natural or synthetic bone is placed in the area of bone loss to promote bone growth.
- **Guided tissue regeneration**. This technique involves inserting a small piece of mesh-like material between the bone and gum tissue. This prevents the gum tissue from growing into the area where the bone should be, allowing bone and connective tissue to regrow.
- **Growth factors**. Proteins that help your body naturally regrow bone may also be used.
- **Soft tissue graft**. In cases where gum tissue has been lost, synthetic material or tissue taken from another area of your mouth is used to cover exposed tooth roots.

FACTORS INFLUENCING TREATMENT SUCCESS

Since each case is different, it is impossible to predict with certainty which grafts will be successful in the long term. Treatment results depend on many factors, including the progression of the disease, how well the patient maintains oral care at home, and certain risk factors like smoking, which may lower the chances of success. Consult with your periodontist to understand the potential level of success in your particular case.[1]

[1] "Periodontal (Gum) Disease—Causes, Symptoms, and Treatment," National Institute of Dental and Craniofacial Research (NIDCR), September 2013. Available online. URL: www.nidcr.nih.gov/sites/default/files/2017-09/periodontal-disease_0.pdf. Accessed April 15, 2024.

Chapter 18 | **Breast Surgeries**

Chapter Contents

Section 18.1 | Surgery Choices for Women with Ductal Carcinoma in Situ or Breast Cancer

If you have ductal carcinoma in situ (DCIS) or breast cancer that can be removed with surgery, you may have options regarding the type of surgery. Often, the choice is between a lumpectomy or other breast-sparing surgery (which removes the cancer but leaves most of the breast) and a mastectomy (which removes the entire breast).

STEPS BEFORE SURGERY

Once diagnosed, treatment will usually not begin immediately. Use this time to:

- Talk with your doctor.
- Get a second opinion.
- Check with your insurance company.
- Learn the facts about your surgery choices.
- Consider what is important to you.

TYPES OF BREAST SURGERY

Most women with DCIS or breast cancer treatable with surgery have three primary options:

Lumpectomy or Other Breast-Sparing Surgery

Breast-sparing surgery involves removing only the DCIS or cancer, some normal tissue around it, and possibly one or more lymph nodes from under the arm. This approach usually allows the breast to maintain its appearance.

After breast-sparing surgery, radiation therapy is often recommended to prevent the cancer from returning to the same breast. Some patients may also require chemotherapy, hormone therapy, or targeted therapy.

Mastectomy

A mastectomy involves removing the entire breast that contains the DCIS or cancer.

There are two main types:

- **Total mastectomy (simple mastectomy).** The entire breast is removed, sometimes along with one or more lymph nodes, using a procedure called "sentinel lymph node biopsy" (SLNB).
- **Modified radical mastectomy.** The entire breast and most of the lymph nodes under the arm are removed. This surgery is rarely used for DCIS.

Radiation therapy, chemotherapy, hormone therapy, or targeted therapy may also be needed after a mastectomy. Post-surgery options include staying flat, wearing a prosthesis, or undergoing breast reconstruction surgery.

Mastectomy with Breast Reconstruction Surgery

Breast reconstruction can be done at the same time as the mastectomy or anytime afterward. A plastic surgeon experienced in breast reconstruction uses an implant or tissue from another part of your body to create a breast-like shape. If the nipple is removed, the surgeon may create a nipple and add a tattoo resembling the areola.

There are two main types of breast reconstruction surgery:

- breast implant
- tissue flap

COMPARING TYPES OF BREAST SURGERY

If you have a choice about which surgery to have, it can be challenging to decide which is best for you. Comparing the different surgeries can help you understand their similarities and differences.

Questions about the Effectiveness of Breast Cancer Surgery

WHICH TYPE OF BREAST CANCER SURGERY IS BEST FOR MY CANCER?

- **Lumpectomy or breast-sparing surgery.** Suitable for most women with DCIS or breast cancer, usually followed by radiation therapy.
- **Mastectomy.** It may be a better choice if you have small breasts with a large area of DCIS or cancer, cancer in more than one part of the breast, or if radiation therapy is not an option.

- **Mastectomy with reconstruction**. Consider if you want breast reconstruction surgery, either simultaneously with the mastectomy or later.

WILL THE TYPE OF SURGERY AFFECT MY LIFESPAN?

Research shows that women who have breast-sparing surgery live as long as those who have a mastectomy, even with reconstruction.

WHAT ARE THE CHANCES OF CANCER RECURRENCE?

- **Lumpectomy or breast-sparing surgery**. There is a chance of cancer returning to the same breast, but this does not usually affect lifespan. About 5–10 percent of women who have breast-sparing surgery with radiation therapy get cancer in the same breast within 12 years.
- **Mastectomy**. Slightly lower chance of recurrence compared to breast-sparing surgery. About 5 percent of women who have a mastectomy get cancer on the same side of the chest within 12 years.
- **Mastectomy with reconstruction**. The chances are the same as for mastectomy since reconstruction does not affect recurrence rates.

RECOVERING FROM BREAST CANCER SURGERY

Pain Management

Most people experience some pain after surgery. Discuss pain control options with your doctor or nurse before surgery, and inform them if pain control measures are ineffective.

Returning to Normal Activities

- **Lumpectomy or breast-sparing surgery**. Most women can return to their usual activities within 5–10 days.
- **Mastectomy**. Recovery may take three to four weeks.
- **Mastectomy with reconstruction**. Recovery depends on the type of reconstruction and can take six to eight weeks or longer.

Potential Post-Surgery Problems

- **Lumpectomy or breast-sparing surgery**. Fatigue and skin changes from radiation therapy.
- **Mastectomy**. Feeling out of balance if you have large breasts and do not have reconstruction, potentially leading to neck and shoulder pain.
- **Mastectomy with reconstruction**. Possible dissatisfaction with the appearance of the new breast shape, pain from hardened implants, or the need for additional surgeries.

ADDITIONAL TREATMENTS AFTER BREAST SURGERY

- **Radiation therapy**. Often required after lumpectomy or breast-sparing surgery. Mastectomy patients may also need it.
- **Chemotherapy, hormone therapy, or targeted therapy**. They may be needed regardless of the type of surgery.

ADDITIONAL SURGERIES

- **Lumpectomy or breast-sparing surgery**. Additional surgery may be needed if cancer cells remain at the edge of the removed tissue.
- **Mastectomy**. Additional surgery may be required if problems arise.
- **Mastectomy with reconstruction**. Likely to need more than one surgery to complete reconstruction.

BODY IMAGE AND QUALITY OF LIFE

- **Lumpectomy or breast-sparing surgery**. The breast should look similar to pre-surgery but may have a small scar.
- **Mastectomy**. The breast and nipple are removed, leaving a flat chest on one side with a scar.
- **Mastectomy with reconstruction**. The new breast will not look or feel like the original or the other.

CONSIDERING WHAT IS IMPORTANT TO YOU

Discuss your options with a breast cancer surgeon, your spouse or partner, family, friends, or other women who have had breast cancer surgery. Consider these questions:

- Am I willing to undergo radiation therapy if I choose lumpectomy or breast-sparing surgery?
- Do I want breast reconstruction surgery if I have a mastectomy?
- Will my insurance cover the procedures I need?
- How important are the appearance and feel of my breast after surgery?

Consider getting a second opinion and talking with others before making a decision about breast cancer surgery.[1]

Section 18.2 | **Breast Biopsy**

WHAT IS A BREAST BIOPSY?

A breast biopsy is a procedure that removes a sample of breast tissue to be checked for signs of disease. A pathologist examines the tissue under a microscope to diagnose breast cancer and other breast diseases. Breast cancer forms in the milk ducts and lobules. Although more common in women, men can also develop breast cancer. Transgender individuals should discuss their risks with their health-care provider.

PURPOSE OF A BREAST BIOPSY

A breast biopsy is the only definitive way to determine if a suspicious change in the breast is cancer. It may be recommended after other tests, such as a physical exam or mammogram, indicate potential breast cancer.

---

[1] "Surgery Choices for Women with DCIS or Breast Cancer," National Cancer Institute (NCI), January 21, 2022. Available online. URL: www.cancer.gov/types/breast/surgery-choices. Accessed July 11, 2024.

REASONS FOR A BREAST BIOPSY

You may need a breast biopsy if:

- You or your health-care provider feels a lump, thickening, or other change in your breast.
- A mammogram, ultrasound, or MRI shows a lump, calcium deposits, or other signs that could indicate cancer.
- The skin on your breast or nipple is red, scaly, or swollen, or your nipple is pulled inward.
- You have abnormal fluid discharge from your nipple.

A biopsy does not mean you have breast cancer; many breast lumps are benign.

TYPES OF BREAST BIOPSY PROCEDURES

There are three main types of breast biopsy procedures, usually done on an outpatient basis:

Fine Needle Aspiration

This biopsy uses a very thin needle to remove a sample of breast cells or fluid and takes about 15 minutes.

Core Needle Biopsy

This biopsy uses a wide needle to remove small tissue samples. Sometimes a vacuum probe is used to gently suction tissue and remove it with a rotating blade. The procedure takes between 15 minutes and an hour.

Surgical Biopsy

Also called an "open biopsy," this surgery removes all or part of a lump and usually takes about an hour.

BREAST BIOPSY PROCEDURE STEPS

Biopsies often use imaging (mammography, ultrasound, MRI, or x-rays) to guide the tissue sample removal.

Fine Needle Aspiration or Core Needle Biopsy Procedure

- The provider cleans the skin and numbs the area with a shot of medicine.
- You may be sitting or lying down, depending on the imaging used.
- For fine needle aspiration, the provider inserts the needle and removes a sample. For core biopsy, a small cut may be made to insert the wide needle or vacuum device.
- Pressure is applied until the bleeding stops.
- The biopsy site is covered with a sterile bandage, and small strips of medical tape may be used to close the wound.

Surgical Biopsy Procedure

- You lie on an operating table, and an IV line may be used to give you medicine to relax.
- The skin over the biopsy area is cleaned.
- Pain is prevented with either a shot of numbing medicine or general anesthesia.
- The surgeon makes a small cut to remove part or all of the lump, sometimes removing surrounding tissue.
- The cut is closed with small strips of medical tape or stitches and covered with a sterile bandage.

PREPARATION FOR THE TEST

Your provider will give you instructions to prepare for the biopsy. If you take blood thinners, including aspirin, you may need to stop taking them. Inform your provider about all medications and supplements you take.

For general anesthesia, you must fast for several hours before surgery. Arrange for someone to take you home if you have general anesthesia or medicine to relax.

RISKS OF THE TEST

Common after-effects include bruising and temporary discomfort. Possible risks include:

- **Infection.** Treatable with antibiotics.
- **Bleeding.** Minor bleeding at the biopsy site.

Your provider will give instructions on caring for the biopsy area and managing discomfort. General anesthesia is generally safe, even for people with other health conditions.

UNDERSTANDING YOUR BIOPSY RESULTS

Results, called a "pathology report," may take several days to a week. The report will include medical terms that your provider can explain. The diagnosis will fall into one of these categories:

- **Normal**. No cancer or abnormal cells are found.
- **Abnormal breast changes (noncancerous)**. Conditions that do not increase cancer risk but may require treatment.
- **Abnormal breast changes (increased cancer risk)**. Cells are not cancerous but increase the likelihood of developing cancer.
- **Breast cancer**. The report will detail the cancer's growth rate, how much the cells resemble normal cells, and other information to plan effective treatment.

Consult a specialist for more information about your biopsy results and potential treatment options.[1]

Section 18.3 | **Breast Implant Surgery**

OVERVIEW OF BREAST IMPLANT SURGERY

Breast implant surgery can be performed in a hospital or surgery center. Depending on the circumstances, patients may need to stay overnight (inpatient surgery) or may be able to go home the same day (outpatient surgery). The procedure can be done under local anesthesia, where the patient remains awake and

[1] MedlinePlus, "Breast Biopsy," National Institutes of Health (NIH), September 28, 2022. Available online. URL: https://medlineplus.gov/lab-tests/breast-biopsy. Accessed July 11, 2024.

only the breast is numbed, or under general anesthesia, where the patient is put to sleep. Most women receive general anesthesia for this surgery. The duration of the surgery can range from one to several hours, depending on the procedure and individual circumstances.

If the surgery is performed in a hospital, the length of the stay will vary based on the type of surgery, any complications, and the patient's general health. Insurance coverage can also affect the length of the hospital stay.

SURGICAL MESH AND BREAST SURGERY

Surgical mesh is typically a flexible, thin sheet made of synthetic materials or from animal- or human-derived tissues called "acellular dermal matrices" (ADM). It is a medical device regulated by the U.S. Food and Drug Administration (FDA). However, the FDA has not cleared or approved any surgical mesh for use with breast implants or in breast reconstruction. Patients should discuss the benefits and risks of mesh with their health-care providers.

SURGICAL CONSULTATION

Before surgery, it is crucial to consult with your surgeon. Prepare to ask questions about the surgeon's experience, the procedure, and expected outcomes. The surgeon should discuss whether you are a good candidate for breast implants, the different types of implants, options for size, shape, surface texture, and placement, and the risks and benefits of implant surgery. Reviewing before-and-after pictures of other patients can help set realistic expectations.

During the consultation, discuss your medical history, including any conditions, drug allergies, previous surgeries, and current medications, including supplements and over-the-counter (OTC) drugs. Inform the surgeon if you think you may be pregnant.

If you are undergoing breast implant surgery for reconstruction, discuss your personal circumstances, such as treatments with chemotherapy or radiation therapy, as these can affect risks and the appearance of the reconstructed breast. The surgeon should also discuss the amount of breast tissue that will remain after surgery and future screening for breast implant ruptures and breast cancer.

Request a copy of the patient labeling for the breast implant. This should include a patient booklet/brochure with important information about the implant, a boxed warning, and a patient decision checklist. Review the patient labeling entirely before surgery.[1]

THINGS TO CONSIDER BEFORE GETTING BREAST IMPLANTS

Before deciding to undergo breast implant surgery, consider the following:

- **Non-lifetime devices.** Breast implants are not lifetime devices. The longer you have them, the more likely it will be for you to have them removed or replaced.
- **Additional surgeries.** You should assume that additional surgeries will be necessary because breast implants are not lifetime devices, and complications can occur.
- **Insurance coverage.** Complications may not be covered by insurance, and the cost of implant removal or replacement might not be covered.
- **Complications and adverse outcomes.** The longer you have breast implants, the more likely you are to experience complications such as capsular contracture, rupture, deflation, wrinkling, asymmetry, scarring, pain, and infection.
- **Monitoring and screening.** Implants need to be monitored for as long as you have them. Regular exams using MRI or ultrasound may be necessary to screen for implant rupture and other complications.
- **Abnormal changes.** If you notice any abnormal changes in your breasts or implants, see your surgeon or health-care provider promptly.
- **Cancer risk.** There is a risk of developing breast implant-associated anaplastic large cell lymphoma

[1] "Breast Implant Surgery," U.S. Food and Drug Administration (FDA), March 8, 2023. Available online. URL: www.fda.gov/medical-devices/breast-implants/breast-implant-surgery. Accessed April 18, 2024.

(BIA-ALCL), a type of non-Hodgkin lymphoma. Treatment involves the removal of the implant and surrounding capsule and possibly chemotherapy and/or radiation therapy.
- **Systemic symptoms**. Some patients report systemic symptoms collectively referred to as "breast implant illness" (BII). Symptoms may reverse with implant removal without replacement.
- **Mesh use in surgery**. Implanting surgical mesh as part of breast implant surgeries has not been approved by the FDA.[2]

RISKS AND COMPLICATIONS OF BREAST IMPLANTS

Some complications and adverse outcomes include:
- **Implant complications**. Breast pain, changes in nipple and breast sensation, additional surgeries, capsular contracture, rupture, deflation, and systemic symptoms.
- **BIA-ALCL**. A type of non-Hodgkin lymphoma.
- **Other cancers**. There have been reports of squamous cell carcinoma (SCC), various lymphomas other than BIA-ALCL, and mesenchymal tumors.
- **Connective tissue disease**. Breast cancer and reproductive problems.
- **Influence on breastfeeding**. Potential effects on breastfeeding and children.

LOCAL COMPLICATIONS

Local complications occurring in at least one percent of breast implant patients include:
- **Asymmetry**. Uneven appearance in size, shape, or breast level.
- **Breast pain**. Pain in the nipple or breast area.

[2] "Things to Consider before Getting Breast Implants," U.S. Food and Drug Administration (FDA), March 8, 2023. Available online. URL: www.fda.gov/medical-devices/breast-implants/things-consider-getting-breast-implants. Accessed April 18, 2024.

- **Breast tissue atrophy**. Thinning and shrinking of the skin.
- **Calcification/calcium deposits**. Hard lumps mistaken for cancer during mammography.
- **Capsular contracture**. Tightening of the tissue capsule around the implant.
- **Chest wall deformity**. Deformation of the chest wall or rib cage.
- **Deflation**. Leakage of saline solution from a saline-filled breast implant.
- **Delayed wound healing**. Prolonged healing of the incision site.
- **Extrusion**. Skin breakdown with the implant appearing through the skin.
- **Hematoma**. Collection of blood near the surgical site.
- **Iatrogenic injury/damage**. Injury or damage to tissue or implant from surgery.
- **Infection**. Occurs when wounds are contaminated with microorganisms.
- **Inflammation/irritation**. Redness, swelling, warmth, pain, and loss of function.
- **Lymphedema/lymphadenopathy**. Swollen or enlarged lymph nodes.
- **Malposition/displacement**. Implant not in the correct position.
- **Necrosis**. Dead skin or tissue around the breast.
- **Nipple/breast sensation changes**. Increased or decreased sensation.
- **Palpability**. The implant can be felt through the skin.
- **Ptosis**. Breast sagging due to aging, pregnancy, or weight loss.
- **Redness/bruising**. Bleeding causing temporary skin color change.
- **Rupture**. Tear or hole in the implant's outer shell.
- **Seroma**. Fluid collection around the implant.
- **Skin rash**. Rash on or around the breast.
- **Unsatisfactory style/size**. Dissatisfaction with the implant's look.

- **Visibility**. Implant visible through the skin.
- **Wrinkling/rippling**. Wrinkling felt or seen through the skin.

ADDITIONAL SURGERIES

Breast implants are not lifetime devices, and complications may require more surgeries. Types of reoperation procedures include:

- **Implant removal**. With or without replacement.
- **Capsulectomy**. Removal or release of scar tissue around the implant.
- **Scar or wound revision**. Removal of excess scar tissue.
- **Hematoma drainage**. Draining blood collections.
- **Implant repositioning**. Correcting implant placement.
- **Biopsy/cyst removal**. Removing lumps through needle or surgical methods.

Breast implant surgery involves significant considerations and potential risks. Thoroughly discuss your options, medical history, and concerns with your surgeon. Be informed about the type of implants, surgical methods, potential complications, and the need for ongoing monitoring and possible future surgeries. Always review and understand the patient labeling and informed consent documents provided by your surgeon.[3]

Section 18.4 | **Breast Reconstruction**

WHAT IS BREAST RECONSTRUCTION?

Many women who have a mastectomy—surgery to remove an entire breast to treat or prevent breast cancer—have the option of having the shape of the removed breast rebuilt.

[3] "Risks and Complications of Breast Implants," U.S. Food and Drug Administration (FDA), December 15, 2023. Available online. URL: www.fda.gov/medical-devices/breast-implants/risks-and-complications-breast-implants. Accessed April 18, 2024.

Women who choose to have their breasts rebuilt have several options. They can be rebuilt using implants (saline or silicone), autologous tissue (tissue from elsewhere in the body), or both implants and autologous tissue.

Surgery to reconstruct the breasts can be done (or started) at the time of the mastectomy (called "immediate reconstruction") or after the mastectomy incisions have healed and breast cancer therapy has been completed (called "delayed reconstruction"). Delayed reconstruction can happen months or even years after the mastectomy.

In the final stage of breast reconstruction, a nipple and areola may be recreated on the reconstructed breast if these were not preserved during the mastectomy.

Sometimes, breast reconstruction surgery includes surgery on the other, or contralateral, breast so that the two breasts will match in size and shape.

HOW DO SURGEONS USE IMPLANTS TO RECONSTRUCT A WOMAN'S BREAST?

Implants are inserted underneath the skin or chest muscle following the mastectomy (Most mastectomies are performed using a technique called "skin-sparing mastectomy," in which much of the breast skin is saved for use in reconstructing the breast.).

Implants are usually placed as part of a two-stage procedure:

- In the first stage, the surgeon places a device called a "tissue expander" under the skin that is left after the mastectomy or under the chest muscle. The expander is slowly filled with saline during periodic visits to the doctor after surgery.
- In the second stage, after the chest tissue has relaxed and healed enough, the expander is removed and replaced with an implant. The chest tissue is usually ready for the implant two to six months after the mastectomy.

In some cases, the implant can be placed in the breast during the same surgery as the mastectomy—without using a tissue expander.

Surgeons increasingly use a material called "acellular dermal matrix" as a scaffold or sling to support tissue expanders and implants. Acellular dermal matrix is a mesh made from donated human or pig skin that has been sterilized and processed to remove all cells to eliminate the risks of rejection and infection.

HOW DO SURGEONS USE TISSUE FROM A WOMAN'S OWN BODY TO RECONSTRUCT THE BREAST?

In autologous tissue reconstruction, tissue containing skin, fat, blood vessels, and sometimes muscle is taken from elsewhere in a woman's body and used to rebuild the breast. This piece of tissue is called a "flap."

Different sites in the body can provide flaps for breast reconstruction. Flaps most often come from the abdomen or back, but they can also be taken from the thigh or buttocks.

Depending on their source, flaps can be pedicled or free.

With a pedicled flap, the tissue and attached blood vessels are moved together through the body to the breast area. Because the blood supply to the tissue used for reconstruction is left intact, blood vessels do not need to be reconnected once the tissue is moved. With free flaps, the tissue is cut free from its blood supply. It must be attached to new blood vessels in the breast area using a technique called "microsurgery." This gives the reconstructed breast a blood supply.

Abdominal and Back Flaps

- **Deep inferior epigastric perforators (DIEP) flap**. Tissue comes from the abdomen and contains only skin, blood vessels, and fat, without the underlying muscle. This type of flap is a free flap.
- **Latissimus dorsi (LD) flap**. Tissue comes from the middle and side of the back. This type of flap is pedicled when used for breast reconstruction. LD flaps can be used for other types of reconstruction as well.
- **Superficial inferior epigastric artery (SIEA) flap**. Tissue comes from the abdomen, as in a DIEP flap, but it

includes a different set of blood vessels. It also does not involve cutting the abdominal muscle and is a free flap. This type of flap is not an option for many women because the necessary blood vessels are not adequate or do not exist.

- **Transverse rectus abdominis myocutaneous (TRAM) flap**. Tissue comes from the lower abdomen as in a DIEP flap but includes muscle. It can be either pedicled or free.

Flaps taken from the thigh or buttocks are used for women who have had previous major abdominal surgery or who do not have enough abdominal tissue to reconstruct a breast. These types of flaps are free flaps. With these flaps, an implant is often used as well to provide sufficient breast volume.

Flaps from the Thigh or Buttocks

- **Inferior gluteal artery perforator (IGAP) flap**. Tissue comes from the buttocks and contains only skin, blood vessels, and fat.
- **Profunda artery perforator (PAP) flap**. Tissue, without muscle, that comes from the upper inner thigh.
- **Superior gluteal artery perforator (SGAP) flap**. Tissue comes from the buttocks as in an IGAP flap but includes a different set of blood vessels and contains only skin, blood vessels, and fat.
- **Transverse upper gracilis (TUG) flap**. Tissue, including muscle, that comes from the upper inner thigh.

In some cases, an implant and autologous tissue are used together. For example, autologous tissue may be used to cover an implant when there is not enough skin and muscle left after the mastectomy to allow for expansion and use of an implant.

HOW DO SURGEONS RECONSTRUCT THE NIPPLE AND AREOLA?

After the chest heals from reconstruction surgery and the position of the breast mound on the chest wall has had time to stabilize, a surgeon can reconstruct the nipple and areola. Usually, the new nipple is created by cutting and moving small pieces of skin from the reconstructed breast to the nipple site and shaping them into a new nipple. A few months after nipple reconstruction, the surgeon can re-create the areola. This is usually done using tattoo ink. However, in some cases, skin grafts may be taken from the groin or abdomen and attached to the breast to create an areola during the nipple reconstruction.

Some women who do not have surgical nipple reconstruction may consider getting a realistic picture of a nipple created on the reconstructed breast from a tattoo artist who specializes in three-dimensional (3D) nipple tattooing.

A mastectomy that preserves a woman's own nipple and areola, called "nipple-sparing mastectomy," may be an option for some women, depending on the size and location of the breast cancer and the shape and size of the breasts.

WILL HEALTH INSURANCE PAY FOR BREAST RECONSTRUCTION?

The Women's Health and Cancer Rights Act of 1998 (WHCRA) is a federal law that requires group health plans and health insurance companies that offer mastectomy coverage to also pay for reconstructive surgery after mastectomy. This coverage must include all stages of reconstruction and surgery to achieve symmetry between the breasts, breast prostheses, and treatment of complications that result from the mastectomy, including lymphedema.

Some health plans are sponsored by religious organizations, and some government health plans may be exempt from WHCRA. Also, WHCRA does not apply to Medicare and Medicaid. However, Medicare may cover breast reconstruction surgery as well as external breast prostheses (including a postsurgical bra) after a medically necessary mastectomy.

Medicaid benefits vary by state; a woman should contact her state Medicaid office for information on whether and to what extent breast reconstruction is covered.

A woman considering breast reconstruction may want to discuss costs and health insurance coverage with her doctor and insurance company before choosing to have the surgery. Some insurance companies require a second opinion before agreeing to pay for surgery.

WHAT TYPE OF FOLLOW-UP CARE AND REHABILITATION IS NEEDED AFTER BREAST RECONSTRUCTION?

Any type of reconstruction increases the number of side effects a woman may experience compared with those after a mastectomy alone. A woman's medical team will watch her closely for complications, some of which can occur months or even years after surgery.

Women who have either autologous tissue or implant-based reconstruction may benefit from physical therapy to improve or maintain shoulder range of motion or help them recover from weakness experienced at the site from which the donor tissue was taken, such as abdominal weakness. A physical therapist can help a woman use exercises to regain strength, adjust to new physical limitations, and figure out the safest ways to perform everyday activities.

DOES BREAST RECONSTRUCTION AFFECT THE ABILITY TO CHECK FOR BREAST CANCER RECURRENCE?

Studies have shown that breast reconstruction does not increase the chances of breast cancer coming back or make it harder to check for recurrence with mammography.

Women who have one breast removed by mastectomy will still have mammograms of the other breast. Women who have had a skin-sparing mastectomy or who are at high risk of breast cancer recurrence may have mammograms of the reconstructed breast if it was reconstructed using autologous tissue. However, mammograms are generally not performed on breasts that are reconstructed with an implant after mastectomy.

A woman with a breast implant should tell the radiology technician about her implant before she has a mammogram. Special procedures may be necessary to improve the accuracy of the mammogram and to avoid damaging the implant.[1]

[1] "Breast Reconstruction after Mastectomy," National Cancer Institute (NCI), February 24, 2017. Available online. URL: www.cancer.gov/types/breast/reconstruction-fact-sheet. Accessed April 15, 2024.

Section 18.5 | Surgery to Reduce the Risk of Breast Cancer

Surgical procedures to reduce the risk of breast cancer are critical options for women at high risk. Understanding these procedures, their effectiveness, and their implications can help women make informed decisions about their health.

WHAT KINDS OF SURGERY CAN REDUCE THE RISK OF BREAST CANCER?

Two types of surgery can be performed to reduce the risk of breast cancer in a woman who has never been diagnosed with breast cancer but is known to be at very high risk of the disease.

A woman can be at very high risk of developing breast cancer if she has a strong family history of breast and/or ovarian cancer, a deleterious (disease-causing) mutation in the *BRCA1* gene or the *BRCA2* gene, or a high-penetrance mutation in one of several other genes associated with breast cancer risk, such as *TP53* or *PTEN*.

The most common risk-reducing surgery is bilateral prophylactic mastectomy (also called "bilateral risk-reducing mastectomy"). Bilateral prophylactic mastectomy may involve complete removal of both breasts, including the nipples (total mastectomy), or it may involve removal of as much breast tissue as possible while leaving the nipples intact (subcutaneous or nipple-sparing mastectomy). Subcutaneous mastectomies preserve the nipple and allow for more natural-looking breasts if a woman chooses to have breast reconstruction surgery afterward. However, total mastectomy provides the greatest breast cancer risk reduction because more breast tissue is removed in this procedure than in a subcutaneous mastectomy.

Even with a total mastectomy, not all breast tissue that may be at risk of becoming cancerous in the future can be removed. The chest wall, which is not typically removed during a mastectomy, may contain some breast tissue, and breast tissue can sometimes be found in the armpit, above the collarbone, and as far down as the abdomen—and it is impossible for a surgeon to remove all of this tissue.

The other kind of risk-reducing surgery is bilateral prophylactic salpingo-oophorectomy, which is sometimes called "prophylactic oophorectomy." This surgery involves the removal of the ovaries and fallopian tubes and may be done alone or along with bilateral prophylactic mastectomy in premenopausal women who are at very high risk of breast cancer. Removing the ovaries in premenopausal women reduces the amount of estrogen that is produced by the body. Because estrogen promotes the growth of some breast cancers, reducing the amount of this hormone in the body by removing the ovaries may slow the growth of those breast cancers.

HOW EFFECTIVE ARE RISK-REDUCING SURGERIES?

Bilateral prophylactic mastectomy has been shown to reduce the risk of breast cancer by at least 95 percent in women who have a deleterious mutation in the *BRCA1* gene or the *BRCA2* gene and by up to 90 percent in women who have a strong family history of breast cancer.

Bilateral prophylactic salpingo-oophorectomy has been shown to reduce the risk of ovarian cancer by approximately 90 percent and the risk of breast cancer by approximately 50 percent in women at very high risk of developing these diseases.

WHICH WOMEN MIGHT CONSIDER HAVING SURGERY TO REDUCE THEIR RISK OF BREAST CANCER?

Women who inherit a deleterious mutation in the *BRCA1* gene or the *BRCA2* gene or mutations in certain other genes that greatly increase the risk of developing breast cancer may consider having bilateral prophylactic mastectomy and/or bilateral prophylactic salpingo-oophorectomy to reduce this risk.

In two studies, the estimated risks of developing breast cancer by age 70 years were 55–65 percent for women who carry a deleterious mutation in the *BRCA1* gene and 45–47 percent for women who carry a deleterious mutation in the *BRCA2* gene. Estimates of the lifetime risk of breast cancer for women with Cowden syndrome, which is caused by certain mutations in the *PTEN* gene, range from 25 to 50 percent or higher, and for women with Li-Fraumeni syndrome, which is caused by certain mutations in the gene, from

49 to 60 percent. By contrast, the lifetime risk of breast cancer for the average American woman is about 12 percent.

Other women who are at very high risk of breast cancer may also consider bilateral prophylactic mastectomy, including:

- those with a strong family history of breast cancer (such as having a mother, sister, and/or daughter who was diagnosed with bilateral breast cancer or with breast cancer before 50 years of age or having multiple family members with breast or ovarian cancer)
- those with lobular carcinoma in situ (LCIS) plus a family history of breast cancer (LCIS is a condition in which abnormal cells are found in the lobules of the breast. It is not cancer, but women with LCIS have an increased risk of developing invasive breast cancer in either breast. Many breast surgeons consider prophylactic mastectomy to be an overly aggressive approach for women with LCIS who do not have a strong family history or other risk factors.)
- those who have had radiation therapy to the chest (including the breasts) before the age of 30 years—for example, if they were treated with radiation therapy for Hodgkin lymphoma (Such women are at high risk of developing breast cancer throughout their lives.)

WHAT ARE THE POTENTIAL HARMS OF RISK-REDUCING SURGERIES?

As with any other major surgery, bilateral prophylactic mastectomy and bilateral prophylactic salpingo-oophorectomy have potential complications or harms, such as bleeding or infection. Also, both surgeries are irreversible.

Bilateral prophylactic mastectomy can also affect a woman's psychological well-being due to a change in body image and the loss of normal breast functions. Although most women who choose to have this surgery are satisfied with their decision, they can still experience anxiety and concerns about body image. The most common psychological side effects include difficulties with body appearance, feelings of femininity, and sexual relationships.

Women who undergo total mastectomies lose nipple sensation, which may hinder sexual arousal.

Bilateral prophylactic salpingo-oophorectomy causes a sudden drop in estrogen production, which will induce early menopause in a premenopausal woman (this is also called "surgical menopause"). Surgical menopause can cause an abrupt onset of menopausal symptoms, including hot flashes, insomnia, anxiety, and depression, and some of these symptoms can be severe. The long-term effects of surgical menopause include decreased sex drive, vaginal dryness, and decreased bone density.

Women who have severe menopausal symptoms after undergoing bilateral prophylactic salpingo-oophorectomy may consider using short-term menopausal hormone therapy after surgery to alleviate these symptoms. The increase in breast cancer risk associated with certain types of menopausal hormone therapy is much less than the decrease in breast cancer risk associated with bilateral prophylactic salpingo-oophorectomy.

DOES HEALTH INSURANCE COVER THE COST OF RISK-REDUCING SURGERIES?

Many health insurance companies have official policies about whether and under what conditions they will pay for prophylactic mastectomy (bilateral or contralateral) and bilateral prophylactic salpingo-oophorectomy for breast and ovarian cancer risk reduction. However, the criteria used for considering these procedures as medically necessary may vary among insurance companies. Some insurance companies may require a second opinion or a letter of medical necessity from the health-care provider before approving coverage of any surgical procedure. A woman who is considering prophylactic surgery to reduce her risk of breast and/or ovarian cancer should discuss insurance coverage issues with her doctor and insurance company before choosing to have the surgery.

The Women's Health and Cancer Rights Act (WHCRA), enacted in 1999, requires most health plans that offer mastectomy coverage to also pay for breast reconstruction surgery after mastectomy.

WHO SHOULD A WOMAN TALK TO WHEN CONSIDERING SURGERY TO REDUCE HER RISK OF BREAST CANCER?

The decision to have any surgery to reduce the risk of breast cancer is a major one. A woman who is at high risk of breast cancer may wish to get a second opinion on risk-reducing surgery as well as on alternatives to surgery.

A woman who is considering prophylactic mastectomy may also want to talk with a surgeon who specializes in breast reconstruction. Other health-care professionals, including a breast health specialist, medical social worker, cancer clinical psychologist, or psychiatrist, can also help a woman consider her options for reducing her risk of breast cancer.

Many factors beyond the risk of disease itself may influence a woman's decision about undergoing risk-reducing surgery. For example, for women who have been diagnosed with cancer in one breast, these factors can include distress about the possibility of having to go through cancer treatment a second time and the worry and inconvenience associated with long-term breast surveillance. For this reason, women who are considering risk-reducing surgery may want to talk with other women who have considered or had the procedure. Support groups can help connect women with others who have had similar cancer experiences.

Finally, if a woman has a strong family history of breast cancer, ovarian cancer, or both, she and other members of her family may want to obtain genetic counseling services. A genetic counselor or other health-care provider trained in genetics can review the family's risks of disease and help family members obtain genetic testing for mutations in cancer-predisposing genes, if appropriate.[1]

[1] "Surgery to Reduce the Risk of Breast Cancer," National Cancer Institute (NCI), August 12, 2013. Available online. URL: www.cancer.gov/types/breast/risk-reducing-surgery-fact-sheet. Accessed April 15, 2024.

Chapter 19 | Cardiac Devices and Procedures

DEFIBRILLATORS

Defibrillators restore a normal heartbeat by sending an electric pulse or shock to the heart. They are used to prevent or correct arrhythmia, a heartbeat that is uneven or too fast. Defibrillators can also restore a heartbeat if the heart suddenly stops pumping blood due to ventricular fibrillation.

Different types of defibrillators work in different ways. Automated external defibrillators (AEDs), found in many public spaces, are designed to save the lives of people who experience cardiac arrest. Even untrained bystanders can use these devices in an emergency. Other defibrillators can prevent sudden death among people at high risk of life-threatening arrhythmias. These include implantable cardioverter defibrillators (ICDs), which are surgically placed inside the body, and wearable cardioverter defibrillators (WCDs), which rest outside the body. ICDs typically consist of a small generator (such as a long-lasting battery) placed under the skin and leads or wires from the generator through the blood vessels to the heart muscle chambers. Adjusting to living with a defibrillator can take time and effort, and it is important to be aware of possible risks and complications.

Defibrillators are used for:

- arrhythmias
- atrial fibrillation (AF)
- cardiac arrest
- congenital heart defects (CHDs)
- heart attack
- heart failure
- sarcoidosis

PACEMAKERS

A pacemaker is a small device that sends electrical pulses to help the heart beat at a normal rate and rhythm. Pacemakers can also help heart chambers beat in sync, improving the heart's efficiency in pumping blood. You may need a temporary (short-term) or permanent (long-term) pacemaker. Permanent pacemakers consist of a small battery implanted under the skin and one or more leads or wires from the battery to the heart muscle chambers.

Pacemakers are used for:

- arrhythmias
- atrial fibrillation
- cardiac arrest
- cardiomyopathy
- congenital heart defects
- heart failure

VENTRICULAR ASSIST DEVICE

A ventricular assist device (VAD) is a mechanical pump that helps the heart pump blood through the body when it cannot pump enough blood on its own. These devices can support the function of the left, right, or both heart ventricles. A VAD includes tubes to carry blood out of the heart and to the blood vessels, a power source, and a control unit that monitors the device's function. This type of heart pump may be used to support the heart until it can pump on its own again while waiting for a heart transplant or to help the heart work better if not eligible for a transplant.

Surgery is required to connect the VAD to the heart. During the surgery, the patient is placed on a heart-lung machine. The pump is placed in the upper part of the belly wall, and tubes connect the pump to the heart and a major artery. After surgery, recovery occurs in the intensive care unit (ICU), and the hospital stay can last two to eight weeks. Patients must follow strict hygiene practices to prevent infection and take anticlotting medications to prevent blood clots.

VADs are used for:

- arrhythmias
- cardiogenic shock
- heart failure

CARDIOVERSION

Cardioversion is a procedure that uses external electric shocks to restore a normal heart rhythm. It is called "defibrillation" when performed in an emergency to prevent death from irregular heartbeats in the ventricles causing cardiac arrest. Scheduled cardioversion procedures treat arrhythmias in the upper chambers of the heart and are performed in hospitals or health-care facilities by cardiologists.

During the procedure, the patient is given anesthesia, and electrodes are placed on the chest and possibly the back. The machine sends brief, low-energy shocks to restore normal rhythm. Recovery involves monitoring heart rhythm and blood pressure for a few hours post-procedure.

Cardioversion is used for:

- arrhythmias
- atrial fibrillation

PERCUTANEOUS CORONARY INTERVENTION

Percutaneous coronary intervention (PCI), or coronary angioplasty, is a nonsurgical procedure that improves blood flow to the heart by opening blood vessels narrowed or blocked by plaque buildup. PCI is commonly used during a heart attack to open a blocked artery. The procedure involves inserting a catheter through blood vessels to the heart, inflating a balloon to open the artery, and often placing a stent to keep the artery open.

Recovery includes monitoring for complications and taking prescribed anticlotting medications. Serious complications are rare but can include bleeding, blood vessel damage, and heart attack.

PCI is used for:

- angina (chest pain)
- atherosclerosis
- coronary heart disease
- heart attack
- overweight and obesity

HEART SURGERY

Heart surgery corrects problems with the heart and surrounding blood vessels when other treatments are ineffective. Traditional heart surgery, or open-heart surgery, involves using a heart-lung machine to circulate blood while the heart is stopped. Some surgeries can now be performed while the heart is still beating (off-pump surgery). Risks are higher in emergency situations or if the patient has other health conditions.

Heart surgery is used for:

- aortic aneurysm
- arrhythmias
- coronary heart disease
- heart attack
- heart failure
- heart valve diseases

STENTS

A stent is a small mesh tube that holds open passages in the body, such as weak or narrow arteries. Stenting is minimally invasive and often follows a cardiac catheterization procedure. After receiving a stent, patients may need anticlotting or antiplatelet medications to prevent complications like blood clots.

Stents are used for:

- aortic aneurysm
- atherosclerosis
- coronary heart disease
- heart attack
- peripheral artery disease (PAD)

CATHETER ABLATION

Catheter ablation stops abnormal electrical signals in the heart that cause arrhythmias. The procedure involves guiding catheters through blood vessels to the heart, where electrodes locate the source of the abnormal signals. Radiofrequency waves, extreme cold, or laser light create a scar to prevent irregular heartbeats.

Risks include bleeding, infection, and a very slight risk of cancer from radiation.

Catheter ablation is used for:

- arrhythmias
- atrial fibrillation
- cardiac arrest
- stroke

CORONARY ARTERY BYPASS GRAFTING

Coronary artery bypass grafting (CABG) improves blood flow to the heart muscle by creating new paths for blood to flow around narrowed or blocked coronary arteries. The surgeon uses a healthy blood vessel from another part of the body to bypass the blockage. CABG can reduce complications for people with obstructive coronary artery disease.

CABG is used for:

- cardiac arrest
- coronary heart disease
- heart attack
- heart failure

TRANSCATHETER AORTIC VALVE REPLACEMENT

Transcatheter aortic valve replacement (TAVR) replaces a faulty aortic valve with an artificial one using a cardiac catheter. TAVR is less invasive than open-heart surgery and is recommended for patients at high risk for traditional surgery.

TAVR is used for:

- congenital heart defects
- coronary heart disease
- heart failure
- heart inflammation
- heart valve diseases[1]

---

[1] "Heart Treatments," National Heart, Lung, and Blood Institute (NHLBI), March 24, 2022. Available online. URL: www.nhlbi.nih.gov/health/heart-treatments-procedures. Accessed April 22, 2024.

Chapter 20 | **Joint, Bone, and Spine Surgeries**

Chapter Contents

WHAT IS JOINT REPLACEMENT SURGERY?

Joint replacement surgery is a procedure where a surgeon removes a damaged joint and replaces it with an artificial part. A joint is where two or more bones come together, such as the knee, hip, and shoulder. The surgery is usually performed by an orthopedic surgeon. Sometimes, only the damaged parts of the joint are replaced or fixed rather than the whole joint.

Joint replacement can relieve pain and improve movement, enhancing overall quality of life (QOL). Hips and knees are the most commonly replaced joints, but shoulders, fingers, ankles, and elbows can also be replaced.

WHAT CAN HAPPEN TO JOINTS?

Joints can be damaged by arthritis, diseases, injuries, or other causes. Arthritis or years of use may cause the joint to wear away, resulting in pain, stiffness, and swelling. Damage inside a joint can limit blood flow, which affects the health, growth, and repair of bones.

WHAT IS A NEW JOINT LIKE?

A new joint, called a "prosthesis," can be made of metal, plastic, or ceramic parts. It may be cemented into place or left uncemented, allowing the bone to grow into it. Both methods may be combined to secure the new joint. Your doctor will discuss the best options with you.

WHEN SHOULD JOINT REPLACEMENT BE CONSIDERED?

Joint replacement surgery may be recommended when other treatments, such as walking aids, physical therapy, medications, exercise, and weight loss, are ineffective in relieving pain and improving movement. Surgery is often considered if you have constant pain and difficulty with daily activities such as walking, climbing stairs, and bathing.

WHAT HAPPENS DURING SURGERY?

The surgical team will administer anesthesia to block pain either in one part of the body (regional anesthesia) or put you to sleep (general anesthesia). The damaged joint will then be replaced with an artificial joint.

The duration of the surgery depends on the extent of joint damage and the surgical method used. Your doctor or a team member will inform you how to prepare for surgery, the duration, and what to expect post-surgery.

WHAT HAPPENS AFTER SURGERY?

The recovery timeline depends on the type of surgery, your medical history, and your support network at home. Temporary pain in the new joint is common as your muscles are weak and your body heals. Pain can bc managed with medications and should subside within a few weeks or months.

Physical therapy helps strengthen the muscles around the new joint and regain motion. As you move your new joint and strengthen your muscles, pain will decrease, flexibility will increase, and movement will improve.

ARE THERE RISKS ASSOCIATED WITH JOINT REPLACEMENT?

All surgeries carry risks, which depend on your overall health, joint health before surgery, and the type of surgery. Post-surgery, it is important to follow your doctor's advice on diet, medication, and exercise. Discuss any pain or movement issues with your doctor.

Joint replacement is usually successful. When problems occur, they are often treatable. Possible complications include:

- infection
- blood clots
- loosening of the new joint
- nerve and blood vessel injuries[1]

---

[1] "Joint Replacement Surgery: Health Information Basics for You and Your Family," National Institute of Arthritis and Musculoskeletal and Skin Diseases (NIAMS), May 2023. Available online. URL: www.niams.nih.gov/community-outreach-initiative/understanding-joint-health/joint-replacement-surgery. Accessed April 22, 2024.

Section 20.2 | Hip Replacement Surgery

WHAT IS HIP REPLACEMENT SURGERY?

Hip replacement surgery, or hip arthroplasty, is a surgical procedure in which an orthopedic surgeon removes the diseased parts of the hip joint and replaces them with artificial parts that mimic the function of the normal hip joint.

You may need hip replacement surgery if you have a disease such as:

- arthritis, including osteoarthritis and rheumatoid arthritis
- osteonecrosis, which occurs when parts of a bone die due to decreased blood supply

Hip replacement surgery may also be necessary if you fracture your hip from an injury, such as a fall, or from a bone disease.

The hip joint is a ball-and-socket joint, one of the largest joints in the body. The upper end of the femur (thighbone) meets the pelvis to create the joint. The ball at the end of the femur is called the "femoral head," and it fits into the socket (acetabulum) in the pelvis.

GOALS OF HIP REPLACEMENT SURGERY

The goals of hip replacement surgery include:

- relieving pain from the damaged or diseased hip joint
- improving the function of the hip joint
- increasing mobility

THE HIP REPLACEMENT PROCEDURE

During a hip replacement, the surgeon makes an incision over the thigh and removes the diseased or damaged bone and cartilage from the hip joint. The head of the femur and acetabulum are then replaced with artificial parts. Over time, surgeons have learned to perform hip replacement with smaller incisions to limit trauma to the soft tissues.

The main parts of most hip replacements that fit against the bone, the socket, and the stem are made of metal. The joint surface (bearing surface) may be made of metal, ceramic, or plastic. Surgeons may use a combination of artificial pieces to replace the hip joint, such as:

- metal ball with a plastic socket lining
- ceramic ball with a plastic socket lining
- ceramic ball with a ceramic socket or lining

Due to complications that may develop, surgeons rarely use metal-on-metal artificial bearing surfaces.

The surgeon will choose pieces that attach differently to the remaining bone, which include:

- **Cemented replacements**. Fasten artificial parts to healthy bones with special glue or cement.
- **Uncemented replacements**. Use artificial parts with a porous surface or another type of surface, allowing bone to grow into the pores to hold the new parts in place. As it takes time for natural bone to grow and attach to the prosthesis, activity may be limited for several months after surgery.
- **Hybrid replacements**. Use a cemented femur part and an uncemented acetabular part.

WHEN IS HIP REPLACEMENT SURGERY NEEDED?

Hip replacement surgery is typically needed to repair damage to the hip joint caused by:

- osteoarthritis
- rheumatoid arthritis
- osteonecrosis
- injuries or fractures from trauma or disease

Before considering hip replacement surgery, health-care providers may recommend other treatments, including:

- pain medications
- physical therapy and exercise programs

- activity changes to limit strain on the hip
- assistive devices such as a cane, crutch, or walker

If these therapies are ineffective in relieving joint pain and limiting activities, the doctor may recommend hip replacement surgery. Technological advances have improved artificial parts, making hip replacement surgery successful for younger individuals.

However, hip replacement surgery may not be recommended for people with certain health conditions. You and your doctor will determine the best treatment based on your health history and the risks associated with the surgery.

PREPARING FOR HIP REPLACEMENT SURGERY

Preparation for hip replacement surgery begins several weeks before the actual procedure. Being as healthy as possible before surgery can aid recovery and lower the risk of complications. Steps to prepare include:

- discussing expectations with your surgeon and health-care team
- performing recommended exercises to strengthen your core, upper body, and leg muscles
- reducing or quitting smoking
- losing weight, if overweight, to decrease the risk of complications
- arranging transportation for the procedure and follow-up visits
- asking for help around the house during recovery
- preparing meals in advance
- setting up a recovery area in your home with essentials within reach

Consider equipment to assist with daily activities, such as:

- safety bars in the bathroom
- raised toilet seat
- shower chair or bench
- assistive devices such as a walker or crutches

WHAT TO EXPECT DURING HIP REPLACEMENT SURGERY

During hip replacement:

- You will receive regional anesthesia (blocking pain in a certain area) or general (putting your whole body to sleep).
- The surgeon will make an incision over the hip, remove the diseased bone tissue and cartilage, and replace the femoral head and acetabulum with artificial parts.
- After surgery, you will be moved to the recovery room.

LIFE AFTER HIP REPLACEMENT SURGERY

Post-surgery, most people experience:

- less pain after recovery
- better mobility
- improved activities of daily living (ADLs) and quality of life (QOL)

Discuss with your doctor safe exercises to increase muscle strength and cardiovascular fitness without injuring the new hip. Avoid high-impact activities such as basketball, jogging, and vigorous tennis to prevent excessive wear or loosening of the new hip.

TIPS TO PREVENT FALLS

- Use a cane or walker if needed for stability.
- Wear supportive shoes with thin nonslip soles; avoid slippers and deep-tread athletic shoes.
- When sidewalks are slippery, walk on grass; in winter, use salt, sand, or kitty litter on icy sidewalks.
- Stop at curbs to check their height before stepping up or down.

PREVENTING FALLS INDOORS

- Keep rooms free of clutter, especially on floors.
- Use plastic or carpet runners on slippery floors.
- Wear supportive shoes with thin nonslip soles indoors; avoid slippers and deep-tread athletic shoes.

- Be mindful of pets to avoid tripping.
- Avoid walking in socks, stockings, or slippers.
- Use skid-proof backing on carpets and area rugs, or tack them to the floor.
- Ensure stairs are well-lit with rails on both sides.
- Install grab bars in the bathroom.
- Use a rubber bath mat or slip-proof seat in the shower or tub.
- Improve lighting in your home; use nightlights or keep a flashlight by your bed.
- Use a sturdy step stool with a handrail and wide steps.
- Keep a cordless phone or cell phone with you to avoid rushing to answer calls. If you fall, you can call for help.
- Consider a personal emergency-response system.

These guidelines will help you prepare for and recover from hip replacement surgery while minimizing risks and improving your QOL.[1]

Section 20.3 | **Knee Replacement Surgery**

WHAT IS KNEE REPLACEMENT SURGERY?

Knee replacement surgery involves replacing parts of the knee joint with artificial components. This procedure is necessary for individuals with severe knee damage that causes significant pain and difficulty performing daily activities, such as walking and climbing stairs. The primary goal of knee replacement is to relieve pain and improve mobility.

Knee replacement surgery is common among older adults but can be performed on individuals of all ages. The decision to undergo surgery depends on overall health and the extent of knee discomfort.

[1] "Hip Replacement Surgery," National Institute of Arthritis and Musculoskeletal and Skin Diseases (NIAMS), August 2023. Available online. URL: www.niams.nih.gov/health-topics/hip-replacement-surgery. Accessed April 22, 2024.

CONDITIONS TREATED BY KNEE REPLACEMENT SURGERY

Knee replacement surgery addresses conditions that cause the cartilage of the knee joint to wear away, including:

- knee osteoarthritis:
  - It often develops over time after an injury or with aging and is the most common reason for knee replacement surgery.
- knee damage from other types of arthritis
- problems from incorrectly formed knee joints

THE KNEE REPLACEMENT PROCEDURE

During the procedure, the surgeon removes damaged cartilage and some bone from the knee joint surfaces. Cartilage covers bones where they meet, providing a smooth surface that helps the bones glide over each other. When cartilage wears away, bones rub against each other, causing pain.

The surgeon attaches artificial parts made of metal and plastic to the bones after removing the damaged cartilage and bone, giving the knee new, smooth surfaces.

Knee replacement surgery can be a total knee replacement, replacing all damaged parts of the knee, or a partial knee replacement, replacing only part of the knee. In a total knee replacement, the surgeon replaces three surfaces:

- end of the shinbone
- end of the thighbone
- back of the kneecap

POST-SURGERY RECOVERY

Some patients go home the same day as the surgery, while others stay in the hospital for a few days. To prevent blood clots, patients often take blood thinners and wear special socks or leg coverings after surgery.

Successful recovery depends significantly on following post-surgery instructions. A physical therapist will teach exercises to strengthen the knee and improve its range of motion. Regular exercise is crucial. Patients may need to use a cane or walker for several weeks and will receive guidance on when they can resume driving.

Most individuals who adhere to recovery instructions can return to nearly all normal daily activities within three to six weeks after surgery.

LIFE AFTER KNEE REPLACEMENT

After recovery, most people experience improved movement and less pain than before surgery. However, an artificial knee is different from a natural, healthy knee. It is important to protect the new knee by:

- maintaining a healthy weight
- engaging in regular physical activity
- avoiding high-impact activities such as jogging, running, and jumping, opting instead for low-impact activities such as walking, biking, and swimming

RISKS OF KNEE REPLACEMENT SURGERY

While the risk of complications is low, possible issues after knee replacement surgery include:

- infection
- blood clots
- heart attack
- stroke
- nerve damage
- scarring that limits knee flexibility

Age, general health, and activity level can influence the risk of complications.

LONGEVITY OF A KNEE REPLACEMENT

A knee replacement typically lasts 15–20 years. After this period, the artificial knee parts may become loose or worn, necessitating another surgery on the same knee.

If considering knee replacement surgery, discuss the risks and benefits with your doctor to determine if the procedure is right for you.[1]

[1] MedlinePlus, "Knee Replacement," National Institutes of Health (NIH), December 26, 2023. Available online. URL: https://medlineplus.gov/kneereplacement.html. Accessed April 22, 2024.

Section 20.4 | **Carpal Tunnel Surgery**

WHAT IS CARPAL TUNNEL SYNDROME?

Carpal tunnel syndrome (CTS) occurs when the median nerve, which runs from the forearm through the wrist into the palm of the hand, becomes pressed or squeezed at the wrist. The median nerve and the tendons that bend the fingers pass through the carpal tunnel—a narrow, rigid tube of ligament and bones at the base of the hand. The median nerve provides feeling to the thumb, index, and middle fingers, and part of the ring finger (but not the little finger). It also controls some small muscles at the base of the thumb.

WHO TREATS CARPAL TUNNEL SYNDROME?

Carpal tunnel syndrome is typically treated by a variety of health-care professionals, including:

- **Neurologists**. Doctors who diagnose and treat nerve disorders.
- **Neurosurgeons**. Physicians who specialize in the diagnosis and surgical treatment of peripheral nerve disorders.
- **Orthopedic surgeons**. Surgeons who specialize in diagnosing and treating injuries to bones, joints, ligaments, tendons, muscles, and nerves.
- **Primary health-care providers**. They include family doctors, internists, and rheumatologists who treat problems as they arise and coordinate care between different specialized health-care providers.

You may also see:

- **Occupational and physical therapists**. Professionals who teach ways to strengthen muscles and joints, minimize pain, and perform activities of daily living (ADLs).
- **Pain management specialists**. Physicians trained in the evaluation and treatment of pain.

- **Physiatrists.** Doctors who specialize in the nonsurgical management of musculoskeletal conditions and can develop a care plan, including rehabilitation.

SURGICAL TREATMENTS FOR CARPAL TUNNEL SYNDROME

Carpal tunnel release is one of the most common surgical procedures in the United States. It involves making a small incision and cutting a ligament to relieve the pressure on the median nerve. Some individuals with CTS may require surgery on both wrists. There are two different methods of carpal tunnel release surgery:

- **Open-release surgery**. This traditional procedure involves making an incision in the wrist and cutting the carpal ligament (the tissue that holds joints together) to enlarge the carpal tunnel. It is generally performed under local anesthesia on an outpatient basis.
- **Endoscopic surgery**. This method involves making one or two small incisions in the wrist and palm. A camera attached to a tube is inserted to view the nerve, ligament, and tendons on a monitor. Using the image as a guide, the surgeon cuts the carpal ligament with a small knife inserted through the tube. This type of surgery may allow for faster recovery and less discomfort than traditional open-release surgery but carries a higher risk of complications and the need for repeat surgery.

Although carpal tunnel surgery may quickly relieve symptoms, full recovery depends on the severity of the CTS and can take months to years. All surgeries carry risks, and some people may experience infections, nerve damage, stiffness, or pain at the scar.

Surgery usually resolves the issue permanently, and it is very rare for CTS to recur after surgery.[1]

[1] "Carpal Tunnel Syndrome," National Institute of Arthritis and Musculoskeletal and Skin Diseases (NIAMS), December 2023. Available online. URL: www.niams.nih.gov/health-topics/carpal-tunnel-syndrome. Accessed April 22, 2024.

Section 20.5 | **Spinal Stenosis Surgery**

WHAT IS SPINAL STENOSIS?

Spinal stenosis occurs when the spaces in the spine narrow, creating pressure on the spinal cord and nerve roots. The spinal cord is a bundle of nerves that runs from the base of the brain down the center of the spine. The nerve roots branch out from the cord. The narrowing usually happens over time and can affect one or more areas of the spine:

- spinal canal:
    - a hollow space in the center of each vertebra (bones in the spine that protect the spinal cord), the spinal cord, and nerve roots run through the spinal canal
- space at the base or roots of nerves branching out from the spinal cord
- openings between vertebrae, through which nerves leave the spine and go to other body parts

There are four regions of the spine:

- cervical spine
- thoracic spine
- lumbar spine
- sacrum and coccyx

Spinal stenosis most commonly develops in the lumbar spine and cervical spine.

WHO TREATS SPINAL STENOSIS?

Doctors who treat spinal stenosis include:

- family or primary care doctors
- neurologists—specialists in disorders and diseases of the spine, brain, and nerves
- neurosurgeons—surgeons who perform procedures for spine, brain, and nerve disorders
- orthopedists—surgeons specializing in bone and joint diseases

- pain specialists—physicians, including anesthesiologists, trained in evaluating, diagnosing, and treating various types of pain
- physiatrists—specialists in physical and rehabilitation medicine
- physical therapists—experts in movement and muscle strengthening
- rheumatologists—specialists in musculoskeletal diseases and autoimmune disorders

SURGICAL TREATMENTS FOR SPINAL STENOSIS

If nonsurgical treatments and medications fail to alleviate symptoms, your doctor may recommend meeting with a surgeon to discuss surgical options. Surgery may be suggested immediately if you experience numbness or weakness that interferes with walking, impaired bowel or bladder function, or other neurological issues.

The decision to undergo surgery depends on:

- the effectiveness of nonsurgical treatments
- the severity of the pain
- other existing diseases and conditions
- overall health
- whether your specific spinal anatomy is suitable for surgery

Not everyone with persistent symptoms is a candidate for surgery. Surgeons will review the risks and potential benefits of the procedure.

TYPES OF SURGERIES FOR SPINAL STENOSIS

Surgeons can relieve pressure on the spinal cord and nerves and restore spine alignment and health through various surgeries, including:

- **Laminectomy**. This surgery involves removing bony spurs and the bone walls of the vertebrae to open up the spinal column and relieve nerve pressure. Doctors may perform a discectomy during a laminectomy, removing part of a herniated disk to relieve spinal cord or nerve root pressure. A facetectomy may also be done, removing part or all of a facet joint to reduce pressure.

- **Spinal fusion**. This surgery treats age-related spine changes and spondylolisthesis by joining two or more vertebrae that have slipped out of their normal position. The surgeon may remove the disk between the vertebrae and use bone grafts or metal devices to secure the bones together.
- **Minimally invasive surgery**. This approach uses smaller incisions than standard surgery, potentially causing less scarring and damage to nearby muscles and tissues, leading to less pain and faster recovery.

POST-SURGERY EXPECTATIONS

Removing and repairing the areas of the spine causing pressure usually helps decrease symptoms. Most people experience less leg pain and improved walking ability after surgery. However, if nerves were severely damaged before surgery, some pain or numbness may persist, or there may be no improvement. Additionally, the degenerative process may continue, and pain or activity limitations may reappear after surgery.[1]

Section 20.6 | **Surgery for Back Pain**

Back pain is one of the most common reasons people see a doctor or miss work. It can affect people of all ages, including school-age children. Back pain can range from a dull, constant ache to sudden, sharp, or shooting pain. It can start suddenly due to an

[1] "Spinal Stenosis," National Institute of Arthritis and Musculoskeletal and Skin Diseases (NIAMS), November 2023. Available online. URL: www.niams.nih.gov/health-topics/spinal-stenosis. Accessed April 15, 2024.

accident or lifting something heavy or develop over time as we age. Insufficient exercise followed by a strenuous workout can also cause back pain.

TYPES OF BACK PAIN

There are two types of back pain:

- **Acute back pain**. Lasts a few days to a few weeks. Most low back pain is acute, resolving on its own within a few days with self-care and without residual loss of function. In some cases, symptoms may take a few months to disappear.
- **Chronic back pain**. Defined as pain continuing for 12 weeks or longer, even after the initial injury or cause has been treated. About 20 percent of people with acute low back pain develop chronic low back pain with persistent symptoms at one year. Chronic pain does not always indicate a serious underlying cause and may persist despite medical and surgical treatments.

TREATMENT FOR ACUTE BACK PAIN

Acute back pain usually improves on its own. Common treatments include:

- Medications:
  - analgesics such as acetaminophen and aspirin
  - nonsteroidal anti-inflammatory drugs (NSAIDs) such as ibuprofen and naproxen (available over the counter and by prescription)
  - muscle relaxants
  - topical pain relief such as creams, gels, patches, or sprays like capsaicin and lidocaine that stimulate nerves in the skin to provide warmth or cold sensations to dull pain
- heat and/or ice to ease pain, reduce inflammation, and improve mobility
- gentle stretching upon advice from a health-care professional

Exercising, bed rest, and surgery are typically not recommended for acute back pain.

TREATMENT FOR CHRONIC BACK PAIN

Chronic back pain is often treated with a stepped-care approach, progressing from simple, low-cost treatments to more aggressive ones, depending on the identified cause. When other therapies fail, surgery may be considered to relieve pain caused by nerve damage, serious musculoskeletal injuries, or nerve compression. Specific surgeries are selected based on individual conditions, but success is not guaranteed, and full recovery can take months with potential permanent loss of flexibility.

SURGICAL OPTIONS FOR BACK PAIN

- **Vertebroplasty and kyphoplasty**. Minimally invasive treatments to repair vertebral compression fractures due to osteoporosis. Vertebroplasty involves injecting bone cement to stabilize the bone, while kyphoplasty uses a balloon to restore vertebral height before cement injection.
- **Spinal laminectomy (spinal decompression)**. Removes bony walls of vertebrae and bone spurs to relieve nerve pressure caused by spinal canal narrowing.
- **Discectomy and microdiscectomy**. Removal of a herniated disc through an incision in the back. Microdiscectomy uses a smaller incision for quicker recovery. Often performed with laminectomy to relieve nerve root pressure.
- **Foraminotomy**. Enlarges the bony hole (foramen) where a nerve root exits the spinal canal, relieving nerve pressure by removing small bone pieces.
- **Nucleoplasty (plasma disc decompression)**. Uses radiofrequency energy to treat mildly herniated discs by vaporizing tissue to reduce disc size and relieve nerve pressure.

- **Radiofrequency denervation**. Uses electrical impulses to interrupt nerve conduction and provide temporary pain relief by heating and destroying target nerves.
- **Spinal fusion**. Joins two or more vertebrae to prevent painful movements using bone grafts and/or metal devices. This procedure may lead to some loss of flexibility, and requires a long recovery period.
- **Artificial disc replacement**. An alternative to spinal fusion for severely damaged discs, replacing the disc with a synthetic one to restore height and movement.
- **Interspinous spacers**. Small devices inserted into the spine to keep the spinal canal open and prevent nerve pinching, used to treat spinal stenosis.

These surgeries aim to relieve pressure on the spinal cord and nerves, restoring spine alignment and health. While most people experience less leg pain and improved mobility post-surgery, some may have lingering symptoms or no improvement if nerves were badly damaged before surgery. The degenerative process may also continue, causing recurrent pain or activity limitations.[1]

[1] "Low Back Pain," National Institute of Neurological Disorders and Stroke (NINDS), March 2020. Available online. URL: www.ninds.nih.gov/sites/default/files/migrate-documents/low_back_pain_20-ns-5161_march_2020_508c.pdf. Accessed April 22, 2024.

Chapter 21 | Gastrointestinal Surgeries

Chapter Contents

WHAT IS APPENDICITIS?

Appendicitis is inflammation of the appendix, a finger-like pouch attached to the large intestine, located in the lower-right area of the abdomen.

COMPLICATIONS OF APPENDICITIS

Untreated appendicitis can cause the appendix to burst, leading to serious complications such as:

- peritonitis—a serious infection that can spread in the abdomen
- appendiceal abscess—an abscess formed due to the burst appendix

TREATMENT OF APPENDICITIS

Doctors typically treat appendicitis by removing the appendix through a surgery called an "appendectomy," performed under general anesthesia in a hospital. Surgery is recommended if there is ongoing or long-lasting abdominal pain, fever, or signs of a burst appendix and infection. Prompt surgery reduces the risk of the appendix bursting and causing further complications.

There are two methods of appendectomy:

- **Laparoscopic surgery**. The surgeon makes a small incision in the abdomen, inserts a laparoscope (a thin tube with a video camera and light), and may make additional small incisions to insert tools to remove the appendix.
- **Open laparotomy**. The surgeon makes a single, larger incision in the lower-right area of the abdomen.

Laparoscopic surgery is becoming more common due to fewer complications, such as hospital-related infections, and a shorter recovery time. The surgeon will recommend the best method based on the patient's condition and medical history.

WHAT IF THE SURGEON FINDS A NORMAL APPENDIX?

If the surgeon finds a normal appendix during surgery, they may still remove it to prevent future appendicitis. Sometimes, surgeons find and correct a different problem during the surgery.

NONSURGICAL TREATMENT OF APPENDICITIS

Patients suspected of having appendicitis are treated with antibiotics before surgery. Some mild cases of appendicitis may be treated with antibiotics alone, although surgery remains the standard of care. Researchers are studying which patients might safely avoid surgery based on symptoms, test results, health, and age.

TREATMENT OF COMPLICATIONS FROM A BURST APPENDIX

The treatment depends on the complication:

- **Peritonitis.** Requires immediate laparotomy to clean the abdomen and prevent infection, followed by appendix removal.
- **Abscess.** The pus is typically drained to allow healing.

COMPLICATIONS AFTER APPENDECTOMY

While generally safe, complications from laparoscopic surgery or open laparotomy can include:

- infection of the surgical site
- abscess formation inside the abdomen
- fistula (an abnormal passage) between the intestine or stomach and the skin
- small bowel obstruction
- ileus (improper bowel function)
- abdominal adhesions (bands of scar-like tissue inside the abdomen)

RECOVERY AFTER APPENDECTOMY

Post-surgery, most patients recover completely from appendicitis without needing to make changes to diet, exercise, or lifestyle. Surgeons usually recommend limiting physical activity for:

- the first three to five days after laparoscopic surgery
- the first 10–14 days after a laparotomy

Discuss the recovery plan with the surgeon to ensure proper healing and return to normal activities.[1]

Section 21.2 | Gallstone Surgery

WHAT ARE GALLSTONES?

Gallstones are hard, pebble-like materials, usually made of cholesterol or bilirubin, that form in the gallbladder. Gallstones can range in size from a grain of sand to a golf ball. The gallbladder can produce one large gallstone, hundreds of tiny stones, or both small and large stones.

When gallstones block the bile ducts of the biliary tract, they can cause sudden pain in the upper right abdomen. This pain is known as a "gallbladder attack" or "biliary colic." If untreated, gallstones can lead to serious complications. However, most gallstones do not cause blockages and are painless, known as "silent gallstones," which typically do not require medical treatment.

TYPES OF GALLSTONES

There are two main types of gallstones:

- **Cholesterol stones**. Usually yellow-green in color, composed mostly of hardened cholesterol. In some countries, cholesterol stones make up about 75 percent of gallstones.
- **Pigment stones**. Dark in color and made of bilirubin. Some people have a mix of both types of stones.

[1] "Appendicitis," National Institute of Diabetes and Digestive and Kidney Diseases (NIDDK), July 2021. Available online. URL: www.niddk.nih.gov/health-information/digestive-diseases/appendicitis. Accessed April 22, 2024.

COMPLICATIONS OF GALLSTONES

Complications of gallstones can include:

- inflammation of the gallbladder
- severe damage to or infection of the gallbladder, bile ducts, or liver
- gallstone pancreatitis, which is inflammation of the pancreas due to a gallstone blockage

Many people do not experience symptoms of gallstones until complications arise. If left untreated, gallstones can be deadly. Treatment usually involves gallstone surgery.

TREATMENT OF GALLSTONES

If gallstones do not cause symptoms, treatment is typically unnecessary. However, if a gallbladder attack or other symptoms occur, it is important to contact a doctor. Symptoms may subside but can reoccur, necessitating treatment. Doctors may refer patients to a gastroenterologist or surgeon for treatment.

The usual treatment for gallstones is surgery to remove the gallbladder (cholecystectomy). In some cases, nonsurgical treatments can treat cholesterol stones, but pigment stones usually require surgery.

Surgical Treatment

Surgery to remove the gallbladder is called a "cholecystectomy" and is one of the most common operations performed on adults in the United States. The gallbladder is not essential, meaning you can live normally without it. General anesthesia is typically administered for the surgery. Once the gallbladder is removed, bile flows directly from the liver through the hepatic duct and common bile duct into the duodenum.

There are two types of cholecystectomy:

- **Laparoscopic cholecystectomy**. Most surgeons perform this type using laparoscopy. It is often an outpatient procedure, allowing patients to go home the same day. Recovery typically takes about a week.

- **Open cholecystectomy**. Used when the gallbladder is severely inflamed, infected, or scarred from previous operations, or if complications arise during laparoscopic surgery. Recovery may require a hospital stay of up to a week, and normal physical activity can resume after about a month.

Some individuals may experience softer and more frequent stools post-surgery due to the continuous flow of bile into the duodenum. These changes are usually temporary but should be discussed with a doctor. Gallbladder surgery complications are rare, with bile duct injury being the most common, which may require additional operations to repair.

Nonsurgical Treatments

Nonsurgical treatments are used in special situations, such as when a patient has cholesterol stones, and a serious medical condition prevents surgery. These treatments can dissolve or break up cholesterol gallstones, but stones may recur, requiring long-term or lifelong treatment.

Types of nonsurgical treatments include:

- **Endoscopic retrograde cholangiopancreatography (ERCP)**. It is used to remove a gallstone stuck in the common bile duct.
- **Oral dissolution therapy**. Medications like ursodiol (Actigall) and chenodiol (Chenix) contain bile acids that break up small cholesterol stones, requiring months or years of treatment.
- **Shock wave lithotripsy**. It uses shock waves to blast gallstones into small pieces. It is rarely used and sometimes in combination with ursodiol.

These treatments offer alternatives for patients who cannot undergo surgery, although the risk of recurrence remains.[1]

[1] "Gallstones," National Institute of Diabetes and Digestive and Kidney Diseases (NIDDK), November 2017. Available online. URL: www.niddk.nih.gov/health-information/digestive-diseases/gallstones. Accessed April 15, 2024.

Section 21.3 | Hernia Surgery

WHAT IS A HERNIA?

A hernia occurs when an organ, intestine, or fatty tissue squeezes through a hole or a weak spot in the surrounding muscle or connective tissue. Hernias often occur at the abdominal wall and can sometimes be visible as an external bulge, particularly when straining or bearing down.

TYPES OF HERNIAS

The most common types of hernias are:

- **Inguinal**. It occurs in the inner groin.
- **Femoral**. It occurs in the upper thigh/outer groin.
- **Incisional**. It occurs through an incision or scar in the abdomen.
- **Ventral**. It occurs in the general abdominal/ventral wall.
- **Umbilical**. It occurs at the belly button.
- **Hiatal**. It occurs inside the abdomen, along the upper stomach/diaphragm.

SURGICAL TREATMENT OPTIONS FOR HERNIAS

Hernia repairs are common procedures, with about 1 million performed each year in the United States. Surgical options include:

- **Laparoscopic repair**. The surgeon makes several small incisions in the abdomen to insert surgical tools and repair the hernia. This can be done with or without surgical mesh.
- **Robotic repair**. It is similar to laparoscopic surgery, but robotic-assisted devices provide ergonomic benefits and technological advancements, such as motion scaling, tremor reduction, and improved optics.
- **Open repair**. The surgeon makes an incision near the hernia and repairs the weak muscle area. This can be done with or without surgical mesh. Open repair using

sutures without mesh is called "primary closure" and is commonly used for inguinal hernias in infants, small hernias, and strangulated or infected hernias.

SURGICAL MESH

Surgical mesh is a medical device used to provide additional support to weakened or damaged tissue. Most surgical mesh devices are made from synthetic materials or animal tissue.

- **Synthetic mesh**. It can be knitted or nonknitted and made from absorbable, nonabsorbable, or a combination of materials.
- **Animal-derived mesh**. It is made from processed and disinfected animal tissue, usually pigs (porcine) or cows (bovine). These meshes are absorbable.
- **Nonabsorbable mesh**. It remains in the body indefinitely and provides permanent reinforcement.
- **Absorbable mesh**. The body gradually absorbs it, and it is not intended for long-term reinforcement. New tissue growth is expected to provide strength as the material is absorbed.

Benefits of Surgical Mesh in Hernia Repair Surgery

Hernias are highly likely to recur, and surgical mesh is often used to strengthen the repair and reduce recurrence rates. Most hernia repairs in the United States use mesh, which has been shown to decrease the likelihood of recurrence and improve patient outcomes through decreased operative and recovery times. However, the suitability of surgical mesh depends on the patient's specific circumstances.

Risks of Surgical Mesh in Hernia Repair Surgery

According to the FDA, the most common adverse events for all hernia repairs—with or without mesh—include:

- pain
- infection
- hernia recurrence

- adhesion (scar-like tissue sticking tissues together)
- obstruction (blockage of the large or small intestine)
- bleeding
- fistula (an abnormal connection between organs, vessels, or intestines)
- seroma (fluid build-up at the surgical site)
- perforation (hole in neighboring tissues or organs)

For hernia repairs with mesh, additional risks include:

- migration of the mesh
- shrinkage (contraction) of the mesh

These complications can be more likely with mesh use, so it is important for patients to discuss the risks and benefits with their surgeons to determine the best treatment option.[1]

Section 21.4 | Hemorrhoid Surgery

WHAT ARE HEMORRHOIDS?

Hemorrhoids, also called "piles," are swollen and inflamed veins around the anus or in the lower rectum.

The two types of hemorrhoids are:

- **External hemorrhoids**. They form under the skin around the anus.
- **Internal hemorrhoids**. They form in the lining of the anus and lower rectum.

COMPLICATIONS OF HEMORRHOIDS

Complications of hemorrhoids can include:

- blood clots in an external hemorrhoid

[1] "Surgical Mesh Used for Hernia Repair," U.S. Food and Drug Administration (FDA), July 13, 2023. Available online. URL: www.fda.gov/medical-devices/implants-and-prosthetics/surgical-mesh-used-hernia-repair. Accessed July 8, 2024.

- skin tags (extra skin left behind when a blood clot in an external hemorrhoid dissolves)
- infection of a sore on an external hemorrhoid
- strangulated hemorrhoid (when the muscles around the anus cut off the blood supply to an internal hemorrhoid that has fallen through the anal opening)
- anemia

DIAGNOSTIC PROCEDURES FOR HEMORRHOIDS

Doctors can often diagnose hemorrhoids based on medical history and a physical exam. External hemorrhoids are diagnosed by examining the area around the anus. Internal hemorrhoids require a digital rectal exam and may involve the following procedures to look inside the anus and rectum:

- **Anoscopy**. It uses an anoscope to view the lining of the anus and lower rectum. This procedure is performed during an office visit or at an outpatient center, usually without anesthesia.
- **Rigid proctosigmoidoscopy**. Similar to anoscopy, but it uses a proctoscope to view the lining of the rectum and lower colon. This procedure is performed during an office visit, at an outpatient center, or in a hospital, usually without anesthesia.

Doctors may also diagnose internal hemorrhoids during procedures for other digestive tract problems or routine examinations of the rectum and colon, such as colonoscopy and flexible sigmoidoscopy.

TREATMENT FOR HEMORRHOIDS

Doctors treat hemorrhoids with procedures during office visits, at outpatient centers, or in hospitals.

Office Treatments

- **Rubber band ligation**. It is used to treat bleeding or prolapsing internal hemorrhoids. A rubber band is placed around the base of the hemorrhoid, cutting off its blood supply and causing it to shrivel and fall off within a week.

- **Sclerotherapy**. It involves injecting a solution into an internal hemorrhoid to form scar tissue, cutting off its blood supply, and shrinking the hemorrhoid.
- **Infrared photocoagulation**. It uses a tool that directs infrared light at an internal hemorrhoid, creating heat that forms scar tissue, cutting off blood supply, and shrinking the hemorrhoid.
- **Electrocoagulation**. It sends an electric current into an internal hemorrhoid to form scar tissue, cutting off blood supply, and shrinking the hemorrhoid.

Outpatient Center or Hospital Treatments

- **Hemorrhoidectomy**. It is performed by a surgeon to remove large external hemorrhoids and prolapsing internal hemorrhoids that do not respond to other treatments. This procedure requires anesthesia.
- **Hemorrhoid stapling**. It uses a special stapling tool to remove internal hemorrhoid tissue and pull a prolapsing internal hemorrhoid back into the anus. This procedure also requires anesthesia.

Complications of hemorrhoids may also require treatment.[1]

Section 21.5 | Ostomy Surgery of the Bowel

Ostomy surgery of the bowel changes how intestinal contents leave the body when part or all of the bowel is diseased, injured, or missing. The surgery creates an ostomy, or stoma, by bringing part of the

[1] "Hemorrhoids," National Institute of Diabetes and Digestive and Kidney Diseases (NIDDK), October 2016. Available online. URL: www.niddk.nih.gov/health-information/digestive-diseases/hemorrhoids/all-content. Accessed July 8, 2024.

bowel through the abdominal wall, allowing intestinal contents to exit through this new opening instead of passing through the anus.

ANATOMY OF THE BOWEL

- **Small intestine**. It includes the duodenum, jejunum, and ileum. Most food digestion and nutrient absorption occur here.
- **Large intestine**. It includes the appendix, cecum, colon, and rectum. It absorbs water from stool and changes it from liquid to solid.

WHAT IS A STOMA?

A stoma is a surgical connection between an internal organ and the skin outside the body. In bowel ostomy surgery, a portion of the intestine is brought through the abdominal wall and connected to the skin, forming a stoma, which can be ¾ inch to 2 inches wide. Since a stoma has no muscle, it cannot control the timing or flow of intestinal contents, requiring the use of an ostomy pouch to collect waste.

TYPES OF OSTOMY SURGERY

The most common types include ileostomy, colostomy, and continent ileostomy. Ileoanal pouch surgery usually requires a temporary ileostomy.

- **Ileostomy**. The ileum (end part of the small intestine) is brought through the abdominal wall to create a stoma, bypassing or removing the entire large intestine.
- **Colostomy**. The colon (part of the large intestine) is brought through the abdominal wall to create a stoma, bypassing or removing the intestine below the stoma.

The stoma may be temporary to allow the intestine to heal or permanent if the large intestine and anus are removed or cannot function properly.

- **Continent ileostomy**. Surgeons create an internal pouch from the ileum with a valve, forming a stoma

that can be drained using a catheter. This procedure is less common and performed in specialized medical centers.
- **Ileoanal pouch surgery (IPAA).** It involves removing the large intestine, creating a pouch from the ileum, and attaching it to the anus. A temporary ileostomy is created to allow the pouch to heal.

PREPARATION FOR SURGERY

Preparation involves consulting with a surgeon and an ostomy nurse, who provides information about the procedure, ostomy care, and life adjustments. The nurse and health-care professionals will determine the optimal location for the stoma, usually in the lower abdomen, based on body positioning and the patient's needs.

SURGICAL PROCEDURES

Ostomy surgery is performed under general anesthesia and can be laparoscopic, robotic, or open:

- **Laparoscopic/robotic surgery.** It involves small abdominal incisions for inserting a laparoscope and surgical tools.
- **Open surgery.** It involves a larger incision to access the abdomen.

POST-SURGERY EXPECTATIONS

Most individuals return to their usual activities after ostomy surgery. An ostomy nurse provides ongoing education and support on topics such as managing waste, diet, hydration, and recognizing complications.

POSSIBLE COMPLICATIONS

Complications can vary based on the type of surgery and patient-specific factors. General complications include bleeding and infection.

Other complications may include:

Ileostomy and Colostomy Complications

- stoma complications
  - bleeding
  - tissue death
  - retraction
  - separation
  - hernia
  - prolapse
  - stricture
- skin complications
  - irritation
  - injury
  - infection
- other complications
  - dehydration
  - nutrient absorption issues
  - intestinal obstruction

Continent Ileostomy Complications

- pouch issues
- stoma issues
- valve problems
- intestinal obstruction

Ileoanal Pouch Surgery Complications

- early complications
  - blood clots
  - pelvic sepsis
  - intestinal obstruction
- late complications
  - pouchitis
  - cuffitis
  - stricture

Frequent bowel movements may cause perianal skin irritation, which can be managed with guidance from an ostomy nurse.

WHEN TO SEEK MEDICAL HELP

Contact a health-care professional if you experience unusual symptoms such as changes in stoma appearance, heavy or persistent bleeding, abdominal cramping, severe nausea, or lack of gas or stool passage. Immediate medical attention is required for severe or persistent symptoms.

Discuss potential complications with your health-care team and follow their recommendations for monitoring and managing your condition.[1]

Section 21.6 | Colon and Rectal Cancer Surgery

COLON CANCER SURGERY

Overview of Colon Cancer

Colon cancer is a disease in which malignant (cancer) cells form in the tissues of the colon. The colon is part of the body's digestive system, which removes and processes nutrients from food and helps pass waste material out of the body. The digestive system includes the esophagus, stomach, small intestine, and large intestine. The colon (large bowel) is about five feet long, and together with the rectum and anal canal, makes up the last part of the large intestine.

Surgical Treatment Options for Colon Cancer

Surgery, which involves removing the cancer, is the most common treatment for all stages of colon cancer. The types of surgery include:

- **Local excision**. If the cancer is at a very early stage, it can be removed without cutting through the abdominal wall. A tube with a cutting tool is inserted through the rectum into the colon to remove the cancer. If

[1] "Ostomy Surgery of the Bowel," National Institute of Diabetes and Digestive and Kidney Diseases (NIDDK), June 2021. Available online. URL: www.niddk.nih.gov/health-information/digestive-diseases/ostomy-surgery-bowel. Accessed July 8, 2024.

the cancer is in a polyp, the operation is called a "polypectomy."

- **Colon resection with anastomosis**. If the cancer is larger, a partial colectomy removes it and a small amount of healthy tissue around it. An anastomosis is then performed to sew the healthy parts of the colon together. Nearby lymph nodes are also removed and examined for cancer.
- **Colon resection with colostomy**. If the two ends of the colon cannot be sewn back together, a stoma (an opening) is created on the outside of the body for waste to pass through, called a "colostomy." A bag is placed around the stoma to collect the waste. The colostomy may be temporary or permanent, depending on the extent of the surgery.

After removing all visible cancer during surgery, some patients may receive chemotherapy or radiation therapy to kill any remaining cancer cells. This treatment is called "adjuvant therapy."

ADDITIONAL TREATMENT

- **Cryosurgery**. It uses an instrument to freeze and destroy abnormal tissue. Also called "cryotherapy."[1]

RECTAL CANCER SURGERY

Overview of Rectal Cancer

Rectal cancer forms in the tissues of the rectum, which is part of the body's digestive system. The digestive system includes the esophagus, stomach, and intestines. The colon (large bowel) is the first part of the large intestine, and the rectum and anal canal make up the last part of the large intestine.

[1] "Colon Cancer Treatment (PDQ®)–Patient Version," National Cancer Institute (NCI), April 6, 2022. Available online. URL: www.cancer.gov/types/colorectal/patient/colon-treatment-pdq. Accessed July 8, 2024.

Surgical Treatment Options for Rectal Cancer

Surgery is the most common treatment for all stages of rectal cancer. The types of surgery include:

- **Polypectomy**. If the cancer is in a polyp, it is often removed during a colonoscopy.
- **Local excision**. If the cancer is on the inside surface of the rectum and has not spread into the rectal wall, it is removed along with a small amount of surrounding healthy tissue.
- **Resection**. If the cancer has spread into the rectal wall, the affected section of the rectum and nearby healthy tissue are removed. The lymph nodes near the rectum are also removed and examined for cancer.
- **Radiofrequency ablation**. It kills cancer cells using a special probe with tiny electrodes. The probe can be inserted directly through the skin with local anesthesia or through an incision in the abdomen with general anesthesia.
- **Cryosurgery**. It uses an instrument to freeze and destroy abnormal tissue. Also called "cryotherapy."
- **Pelvic exenteration**. If the cancer has spread to nearby organs, the lower colon, rectum, and bladder are removed. In women, the cervix, vagina, ovaries, and nearby lymph nodes may be removed. In men, the prostate may be removed. Stomas are created for urine and stool to flow into a collection bag.

Post-Surgery Procedures

After removing the cancer, the surgeon will either:

- perform an anastomosis, sewing the healthy parts of the rectum together, or sewing the remaining rectum to the colon or the colon to the anus; or
- create a stoma for waste to pass through if the cancer is too close to the anus, called a "colostomy."

Radiation therapy and/or chemotherapy may be given before surgery to shrink the tumor, make it easier to remove, and help with bowel control after surgery. This is called "neoadjuvant therapy." After surgery, some patients may receive radiation therapy and/or chemotherapy to kill any remaining cancer cells, known as "adjuvant therapy."[2]

Section 21.7 | Surgical Treatment of Esophageal Cancer

SURGICAL RESECTION AND MULTIMODALITY THERAPY

For patients with minimally invasive resectable esophageal cancer, surgical resection alone offers the potential for cure. However, for patients with locally advanced resectable esophageal cancer, therapeutic management has evolved significantly over the past few decades. Due to the risk of distant metastases and local relapse, multimodality therapy that integrates chemotherapy, radiation therapy, and surgical resection has become the standard of care.

PALLIATION OF ESOPHAGEAL CANCER

Effective palliation may be obtained in individual cases with various combinations (see Table 21.1) of the following:

- surgery
- chemotherapy
- radiation therapy
- stents, photodynamic therapy, and endoscopic therapy with Nd:YAG laser

Self-expandable metal stent positioning is the recommended method for palliation of dysphagia from esophageal cancer.

[2] "Rectal Cancer Treatment (PDQ®)–Patient Version," National Cancer Institute (NCI), March 22, 2024. Available online. URL: www.cancer.gov/types/colorectal/patient/rectal-treatment-pdq. Accessed July 8, 2024.

Table 21.1. Treatment Options for Esophageal Cancer

Stage (TNM Staging Criteria)	Treatment Options
Stage 0 Esophageal Cancer	• Surgery • Endoscopic resection
Stage I Esophageal Cancer	• Chemoradiation therapy followed by surgery • Surgery alone
Stage II Esophageal Cancer	• Chemoradiation therapy followed by surgery • Surgery alone • Chemotherapy followed by surgery • Definitive chemoradiation therapy
Stage III Esophageal Cancer	• Chemoradiation therapy followed by surgery • Preoperative chemotherapy followed by surgery • Definitive chemoradiation therapy
Stage IV Esophageal Cancer	• Chemoradiation therapy followed by surgery (for patients with stage IVA disease) • Chemotherapy, which has provided partial responses for patients with metastatic distal esophageal adenocarcinomas • Adjuvant therapy for patients with completely resected (negative margins) esophageal adenocarcinoma, esophageal squamous cell carcinoma, or gastroesophageal junction cancer who had residual pathological disease after concurrent chemoradiation therapy • Immunotherapy and chemoimmunotherapy for patients with previously untreated, unresectable, advanced or metastatic esophageal squamous cell carcinoma • Immunotherapy and chemoimmunotherapy for patients with previously untreated advanced or metastatic esophageal adenocarcinoma or gastroesophageal junction cancer • Immunotherapy for patients who relapse after one prior line of standard therapy • Nivolumab and chemotherapy for patients with adenocarcinoma • Nd:YAG endoluminal tumor destruction or electrocoagulation • Endoscopic-placed stents to provide palliation of dysphagia • Radiation therapy with or without intraluminal intubation and dilation • Intraluminal brachytherapy to provide palliation of dysphagia • Clinical trials evaluating single-agent or combination chemotherapy

Table 21.1. Continued

Stage (TNM Staging Criteria)	Treatment Options
Recurrent Esophageal Cancer	• Palliative use of the other therapies, including supportive care • Immunotherapy and chemoimmunotherapy for patients with recurrent esophageal squamous cell carcinoma

SURGERY

Surgery for Barrett Esophagus

The prevalence of Barrett metaplasia in adenocarcinoma of the esophagus suggests that Barrett esophagus is a premalignant condition. Endoscopic surveillance of patients with Barrett metaplasia may detect adenocarcinoma at an earlier stage, making it more amenable to curative resection. Strong consideration should be given to resection in patients with high-grade dysplasia in the setting of Barrett metaplasia.

Surgery for Esophageal Cancer

The survival rate for patients with esophageal cancer is poor. Surgical treatment of resectable esophageal cancers results in five-year survival rates of 5–30 percent, with higher rates in patients with early-stage cancers. Asymptomatic small tumors confined to the esophageal mucosa or submucosa are detected only by chance. Surgery is the treatment of choice for these small tumors. Once symptoms, such as dysphagia, are present, esophageal cancers usually have invaded the muscularis propria or beyond and may have metastasized to lymph nodes or other organs.

In some patients with partial esophageal obstruction, dysphagia may be relieved by placement of an expandable metallic stent or by radiation therapy if the patient has disseminated disease or is not a candidate for surgery. Alternative methods of relieving dysphagia have been reported, including laser therapy and electrocoagulation to destroy intraluminal tumor.

In the presence of complete esophageal obstruction without clinical evidence of systemic metastasis, surgical excision of the tumor with mobilization of the stomach to replace the esophagus has been the traditional means of relieving dysphagia.

Optimal Surgical Approaches

The optimal surgical approach for radical resection of esophageal cancer is not known. One approach advocates transhiatal esophagectomy with anastomosis of the stomach to the cervical esophagus. Another approach advocates abdominal mobilization of the stomach and transthoracic excision of the esophagus with anastomosis of the stomach to the upper thoracic esophagus or the cervical esophagus. One study concluded that transhiatal esophagectomy was associated with lower morbidity than transthoracic esophagectomy with extended en bloc lymphadenectomy. However, median overall disease-free and quality-adjusted survival did not differ significantly. Similarly, no differences in long-term quality of life (QOL) using validated QOL instruments have been reported.

More recently, minimally invasive approaches have emerged that offer potential advantages of smaller incisions, decreased intraoperative blood loss, fewer postoperative complications, and shorter hospital stays. However, the ability to obtain negative surgical margins, the adequacy of lymph node dissection, and long-term outcomes have not been fully established with this approach.

Considerations for Older Patients

In the United States, the median age of patients presenting with esophageal cancer is 68 years. A retrospective review of 505 consecutive patients operated on by a single surgical team over 17 years found no difference in perioperative mortality, median survival, or palliative benefit of esophagectomy on dysphagia between patients older than 70 years and their younger peers. All patients in this series were selected for surgery based on potential operative risk. Age alone does not determine therapy for patients with potentially resectable disease.[1]

---

[1] "Esophageal Cancer Treatment (PDQ®)," National Cancer Institute (NCI), February 6, 2024. Available online. URL: www.cancer.gov/types/esophageal/hp/esophageal-treatment-pdq#section_4.15. Accessed July 7, 2024.

Chapter 22 | **Understanding Weight-Loss Surgery**

WHAT IS WEIGHT-LOSS SURGERY?

Weight loss surgery, also known as "metabolic and bariatric surgery," encompasses operations that help individuals lose weight by making changes to the digestive system. "Metabolic" refers to how the body gets energy, while "bariatric" relates to treatment for excessive weight.

Some types of weight-loss surgery reduce the stomach size, limiting food and drink intake, so you feel full sooner. Other types alter the small intestine, decreasing calorie absorption. Additionally, weight-loss surgery can affect hormones or bacteria in the gastrointestinal (GI) tract to reduce appetite and improve metabolism.

WHO ARE GOOD CANDIDATES FOR WEIGHT-LOSS SURGERY?

You may be a good candidate for weight-loss surgery if you are an adult with obesity who has not been able to lose excess weight or maintain weight loss through other methods such as diet, exercise, or medications.

Body mass index (BMI) determines eligibility for weight-loss surgery. For individuals with a BMI of 35 or higher, obesity is often difficult to manage with diet and exercise alone, so health-care professionals may recommend surgery. For those with a BMI of 30–35 who have type 2 diabetes that is hard to control with medications and lifestyle changes, surgery may be considered.

Weight-loss surgery may also be an option if you have serious health problems related to obesity, such as type 2 diabetes or sleep apnea. The surgery can improve many medical conditions linked to obesity, particularly type 2 diabetes.

WHAT ARE THE SURGICAL OPTIONS?

The best type of weight-loss surgery depends on several factors, which you should discuss with your doctor. In the United States, surgeons most often perform three types of operations:

- gastric sleeve
- gastric bypass
- adjustable gastric band

A less common procedure is biliopancreatic diversion with a duodenal switch.

Gastric Sleeve

In gastric sleeve surgery, also called "vertical sleeve gastrectomy," a surgeon removes most of the stomach, leaving a banana-shaped section. This reduces the stomach's capacity, making you feel full sooner and potentially affecting hormones or bacteria that influence appetite and metabolism. This surgery is irreversible.

PROS

- greater weight loss than gastric band
- no changes to intestines
- no foreign objects placed in the body
- short hospital stay

CONS

- irreversible
- risk of vitamin and iron deficiency
- higher chance of surgery-related problems than gastric band
- risk of acid reflux and hiatal hernia

Gastric Bypass

Gastric bypass, or "Roux-en-Y gastric bypass," involves three steps.

- First, the stomach is stapled to create a small pouch.
- Second, the small intestine is divided, and the lower part is attached to the stomach pouch, bypassing the

upper part of the small intestine to reduce calorie absorption.
- Third, the upper part of the small intestine is reconnected to allow digestive juices to flow and fully digest food.

This surgery affects GI tract hormones and bacteria, influencing appetite and metabolism. It is difficult to reverse.

PROS
- greater weight loss than gastric band
- no foreign objects placed in the body

CONS
- difficult to reverse
- higher chance of vitamin and iron deficiency
- higher chance of surgery-related problems than gastric band
- may increase the risk of alcohol use disorder

Adjustable Gastric Band

In adjustable gastric band surgery, a ring with an inflatable band is placed around the top of the stomach to create a small pouch. The band is adjustable via a port under the skin. If the band causes problems or is ineffective, it can be removed.

PROS
- adjustable and reversible
- short hospital stay
- no changes to intestines
- lowest risk of vitamin deficiency

CONS
- less weight loss than other types
- requires frequent follow-up visits
- possible future surgery for adjustments or removal

Biliopancreatic Diversion with Duodenal Switch

This mixed surgery involves two procedures: a gastric sleeve followed by a division of the small intestine into two tracts, reducing calorie and nutrient absorption. It results in more weight loss but has higher risks of deficiencies and surgery-related problems, making it less common.

HOW IS THE SURGERY PERFORMED?

Weight-loss surgery is mostly performed laparoscopically, requiring small cuts and using thin tools and a camera. This method has fewer risks, less pain, and quicker recovery compared to open surgery, which may be necessary for some individuals with high obesity or complex medical issues.

WHAT SHOULD YOU EXPECT BEFORE SURGERY?

Before surgery, you will meet with health-care professionals, including:

- internist
- dietitian
- psychiatrist or psychologist
- bariatric surgeon

They will evaluate your medical history, physical condition, and readiness for surgery, and provide guidance on preparing for and adjusting to life after surgery.

WHAT SHOULD YOU EXPECT AFTER SURGERY?

Post-surgery, you will need to rest and recover, gradually increasing physical activity. Your diet will progress from liquids to soft foods and eventually to solid foods, focusing on small, well-chewed meals. You will also need to take prescribed dietary supplements.

HOW MUCH WEIGHT CAN YOU EXPECT TO LOSE?

Weight loss varies by individual and type of surgery. On average, people lose between 38 and 87 pounds in the first year, with gastric bypass often resulting in greater weight loss but more complications.

WHAT ARE THE BENEFITS OF WEIGHT-LOSS SURGERY?

Weight-loss surgery can help you lose weight and improve obesity-related health issues such as:

- type 2 diabetes
- high blood pressure (HBP)
- heart disease
- sleep apnea

It can enhance mobility, mood, and quality of life (QOL) and reduce the need for medications.

WHAT ARE THE SIDE EFFECTS OF BARIATRIC SURGERY?

Side effects may include:

- bleeding
- infection
- leakage
- diarrhea
- blood clots
- nutritional deficiencies

Follow-up procedures may be necessary, and rare complications can be fatal.

Long-term issues may include:

- strictures
- hernias
- changes in alcohol absorption

By understanding these aspects, you can make an informed decision about weight-loss surgery and its potential benefits and risks.[1]

[1] "Weight-Loss (Metabolic and Bariatric) Surgery," National Institute of Diabetes and Digestive and Kidney Diseases (NIDDK), July 2016. Available online. URL: www.niddk.nih.gov/health-information/weight-management/bariatric-surgery. Accessed July 8, 2024.

Chapter 23 | Gynecologic and Obstetric Surgeries

Chapter Contents

Section 23.1 | **Cesarean Delivery**

WHAT IS A CESAREAN DELIVERY?

A cesarean delivery, also known as a "C-section" or "cesarean birth," is the surgical delivery of a baby through an incision in a woman's abdomen and uterus. After the baby is removed, the uterus and abdomen are closed with stitches that dissolve later.

WHEN IS A CESAREAN DELIVERY NEEDED?

Cesarean delivery may be necessary in the following circumstances:

- **Labor is not progressing**. Contractions may not open the cervix enough for the baby to move into the vagina for delivery.
- **The infant's health is in danger**. The umbilical cord may become pinched, or the fetus may have an abnormal heart rate. A cesarean delivery allows for a quicker delivery to address health issues.
- **The baby is in the wrong position**. This includes breech presentation (feet first), transverse (sideways), or oblique (diagonal) positions.
- **Multiple pregnancy**. Cesarean delivery may be needed if labor starts prematurely, if the fetuses are not positioned well for a natural delivery, or if there are other complications.
- **The baby is too large**. Larger infants are at risk for complications during delivery, such as shoulder dystocia.
- **Placenta problems**. Issues such as improper formation or placement of the placenta can cause problems, including restricted oxygen and nutrient flow or vaginal bleeding.
- **Maternal infection**. Conditions like HIV or herpes could be passed to the baby during vaginal birth.
- **Specific medical conditions**. A cesarean delivery may better manage the mother's health issues.

Women undergoing cesarean delivery may receive pain medication through an epidural block, spinal block, or general anesthesia.

WHAT ARE THE RISKS OF A CESAREAN DELIVERY?

As a surgical procedure, cesarean delivery has risks and possible complications for both mother and baby, including:

- infection
- blood loss
- blood clots
- injury to surrounding structures
- reactions to medication or anesthesia

Women may also have a longer hospital stay compared to those who have had a vaginal delivery. Multiple cesarean deliveries increase the risk of uterine rupture and placenta problems in future pregnancies.

CAN A CESAREAN DELIVERY BE REQUESTED?

Some women may request a cesarean delivery even if vaginal delivery is possible. The decision should be made after detailed discussions with a health-care provider, considering the consequences on current and future pregnancies. The safest method of delivery, unless medically necessary, is an uncomplicated vaginal delivery. Delivery should not occur before 39 weeks of pregnancy unless necessary.[1]

HOW IS A CESAREAN DELIVERY DONE?

Before surgery, you will receive pain medication. Options include:

- **Epidural block.** Numbs the lower part of the body through an injection in the spine.
- **Spinal block.** Numbs the lower part of the body through an injection directly into the spinal fluid.

[1] "What Is a C-Section?" *Eunice Kennedy Shriver* National Institute of Child Health and Human Development (NICHD), September 1, 2017. Available online. URL: www.nichd.nih.gov/health/topics/labor-delivery/topicinfo/c-section. Accessed April 15, 2024.

- **General anesthesia**. Makes you unconscious during surgery, often used in emergencies.

During surgery, the surgeon will perform the following:

- Make a cut in the abdomen and uterus.
- Open the amniotic sac and take out the baby.
- Cut the umbilical cord and remove the placenta.
- Close the uterus and abdomen with stitches.[2]

WHAT IS VAGINAL BIRTH AFTER CESAREAN?

Vaginal birth after cesarean (VBAC) refers to the vaginal delivery of a baby after a previous cesarean delivery. Research shows that for many women, attempting vaginal birth after a prior cesarean—known as a "trial of labor after cesarean delivery" (TOLAC)—can be a safe option. Approximately 75 percent of VBAC attempts are successful among appropriate candidates.

WHEN IS VAGINAL BIRTH AFTER CESAREAN APPROPRIATE?

Vaginal birth after cesarean may be safe and appropriate for women who:

- have had a low-transverse uterine incision (the most common type)
- have had two previous low-transverse cesarean incisions
- are carrying twins
- have an unknown type of uterine incision

Benefits of Vaginal Birth after Cesarean

- no abdominal surgery
- lower risk of hemorrhage and infection compared to a C-section
- faster recovery

[2] MedlinePlus, "Cesarean Delivery," National Institutes of Health (NIH), April 20, 2023. Available online. URL: https://medlineplus.gov/cesareandelivery.html. Accessed April 15, 2024.

- avoiding risks associated with multiple cesarean deliveries
- greater likelihood of having more children in the future

If labor fails to progress or other complications arise, a C-section may be needed after attempting TOLAC. Most risks associated with a C-section after TOLAC are similar to those with a repeat cesarean, including:

- uterine rupture
- maternal hemorrhage and infection
- blood clots
- need for a hysterectomy[3]

Section 23.2 | **Hysterectomy**

WHAT IS A HYSTERECTOMY?

A hysterectomy is a surgical procedure to remove a woman's uterus, also known as the "womb." The uterus is where a baby grows during pregnancy. During the surgery, the entire uterus is usually removed. Your doctor may also remove your fallopian tubes and ovaries. After a hysterectomy, you will no longer have menstrual periods and cannot become pregnant.

WHY WOULD YOU NEED A HYSTERECTOMY?

A hysterectomy may be necessary for several reasons, including:

- **Uterine fibroids.** Noncancerous growths in the uterine wall that can cause pain or heavy bleeding.
- **Heavy or unusual vaginal bleeding.** Caused by hormone changes, infection, cancer, or fibroids.
- **Uterine prolapse.** When the uterus slips from its usual place into the vagina, often after multiple vaginal births, menopause, or due to obesity.

[3] "What Is Vaginal Birth after Cesarean (VBAC)?" *Eunice Kennedy Shriver* National Institute of Child Health and Human Development (NICHD), September 1, 2017. Available online. URL: www.nichd.nih.gov/health/topics/labor-delivery/topicinfo/vbac. Accessed April 15, 2024.

- **Endometriosis**. When tissue that normally lines the uterus grows outside it, causing severe pain and bleeding.
- **Adenomyosis**. When the uterine lining grows into the uterine walls, leading to thickening, pain, and heavy bleeding.
- **Cancer or precancer**. Of the uterus, ovary, cervix, or endometrium, where hysterectomy may be the best treatment option.

WHAT ARE SOME ALTERNATIVES TO HYSTERECTOMY?

Hysterectomy is a major surgery and is sometimes medically necessary. However, other treatments may be tried first:

- **Watchful waiting**. For uterine fibroids, which may shrink after menopause.
- **Exercises**. Kegel exercises can help with uterine prolapse by strengthening pelvic muscles.
- **Medicine**. For endometriosis or heavy bleeding, including over-the-counter (OTC) pain relievers, hormonal birth control, or a hormonal intrauterine device (IUD).
- **Vaginal pessary**. A device inserted into the vagina to support the uterus in cases of uterine prolapse.
- **Surgery**. Less invasive options such as laparoscopic surgery for endometriosis, dilation and curettage (D&C) for heavy bleeding, endometrial ablation, myomectomy for fibroids, and uterine artery embolization (UAE) or MR-guided focused ultrasound (MR[F]US) to shrink fibroids.

WHAT ARE THE DIFFERENT TYPES OF HYSTERECTOMIES?

- **Total hysterectomy**. Removal of the entire uterus, including the cervix, with or without the fallopian tubes and ovaries.
- **Partial hysterectomy**. Also called "subtotal or supracervical hysterectomy," removes the upper part of the uterus but leaves the cervix.

- **Radical hysterectomy**. Removal of the uterus, cervix, tissues on both sides of the cervix, and the upper part of the vagina, often used to treat certain cancers.

WILL THE DOCTOR REMOVE YOUR OVARIES DURING THE HYSTERECTOMY?

The decision to remove ovaries during a hysterectomy depends on the reason for the surgery. Removing ovaries lowers the risk of ovarian cancer but can lead to menopause symptoms. Keeping the ovaries may help protect estrogen against conditions like heart disease and osteoporosis. Discuss the risks and benefits with your doctor.

WILL THE HYSTERECTOMY CAUSE YOU TO ENTER MENOPAUSE?

If your ovaries are removed during the hysterectomy, you will experience menopause symptoms immediately. If the ovaries are not removed, you may still enter menopause a few years earlier than the average age.

HOW IS A HYSTERECTOMY PERFORMED?

Hysterectomy can be performed in several ways, depending on your health and the reason for the surgery:

- **Abdominal hysterectomy**. An incision in the lower abdomen.
- **Vaginal hysterectomy**. Performed through a small incision in the vagina.
- **Laparoscopic hysterectomy**. Uses a laparoscope and small incisions in the abdomen.
- **Robotic surgery**. A robotic arm guided by the surgeon through small abdominal incisions.

HOW LONG DOES IT TAKE TO RECOVER FROM A HYSTERECTOMY?

Recovery time varies based on the type of surgery:

- **Abdominal surgery**. Four to six weeks.
- **Vaginal, laparoscopic, or robotic surgery**. Three to four weeks.

WHAT CHANGES CAN YOU EXPECT AFTER A HYSTERECTOMY?

While recovery can take a few weeks, many women experience an improved quality of life (QOL) due to relief from symptoms. Changes may include:

- **Menopause**. No more periods, and if ovaries are removed, menopause symptoms.
- **Sexual feelings**. Possible vaginal dryness or reduced interest in sex, especially if ovaries are removed.
- **Increased risk for other health problems**. If both ovaries are removed, there may be higher risks for bone loss, heart disease, and urinary incontinence.
- **Sense of loss**. Some women may feel grief or depression due to the loss of fertility.

WILL YOUR SEX LIFE CHANGE AFTER A HYSTERECTOMY?

Many women report a better sex life due to relief from pain or heavy bleeding. Menopause symptoms may cause vaginal dryness or reduced interest in sex, but using a water-based lubricant and allowing more time for arousal can help.

DO YOU STILL NEED TO HAVE PAP TESTS AFTER A HYSTERECTOMY?

You may still need regular Pap tests if you did not have your cervix removed or if the hysterectomy was due to cancer or precancer. Consult your doctor for personalized advice.[1]

Section 23.3 | **Uterine Fibroid Surgery**

WHAT ARE FIBROIDS?

Fibroids are muscular tumors that grow in the wall of the uterus (womb). They are almost always benign (noncancerous). While

[1] Office on Women's Health (OWH), "Hysterectomy," U.S. Department of Health and Human Services (HHS), December 29, 2022. Available online. URL: www.womenshealth.gov/a-z-topics/hysterectomy. Accessed July 8, 2024.

many women with fibroids experience no symptoms, those who do often find fibroids hard to live with due to pain and heavy menstrual bleeding. Fibroids can also pressure the bladder, causing frequent urination, or the rectum, causing rectal pressure. If fibroids grow large, they can cause the abdomen to enlarge, making a woman look pregnant. About 20–80 percent of women develop fibroids by age 50, with the highest prevalence in women in their 40s and early 50s.

CAN FIBROIDS TURN INTO CANCER?

Fibroids are almost always benign. Rarely (less than one in 1,000 cases), a cancerous fibroid called "leiomyosarcoma" can occur. These cancers are not thought to arise from existing fibroids. Having fibroids does not increase the risk of developing a cancerous fibroid or other forms of cancer in the uterus.

SYMPTOMS

Most fibroids do not cause symptoms, but some women with fibroids may experience:

- heavy bleeding (which can cause anemia) or painful periods
- a feeling of fullness in the pelvic area
- enlargement of the lower abdomen
- frequent urination
- pain during sex
- lower back pain
- complications during pregnancy and labor, including a six-time greater risk of cesarean section
- rare reproductive problems, such as infertility

DIAGNOSIS

Fibroids are often discovered during a regular pelvic exam. The doctor can feel fibroids as lumps or masses on the uterus. The size of fibroids is sometimes compared to the size of the uterus if the woman is pregnant or to objects like fruits or balls (e.g., grape, orange, walnut, or golf ball).

To confirm the presence of fibroids, imaging tests are used, including:

- **Ultrasound**. It uses sound waves to produce a picture, either through the abdomen or vagina.
- **Magnetic resonance imaging (MRI)**. It uses magnets and radio waves to create detailed images.
- **X-rays**. It uses radiation to view internal structures.
- **Computed tomography (CT) scan**. It takes multiple x-ray images from different angles for a complete view.
- **Hysterosalpingogram (HSG) or sonohysterogram**. It involves injecting dye or water into the uterus and taking x-ray or ultrasound images.

In some cases, surgery may be needed to confirm fibroids:

- **Laparoscopy**. It involves inserting a thin scope with a camera through a small incision near the navel.
- **Hysteroscopy**. It involves passing a scope with a light through the vagina and cervix into the uterus.

SURGICAL TREATMENTS

If you have moderate or severe symptoms, surgery may be the best treatment option. The surgical options include:

Myomectomy

Myomectomy involves removing fibroids while preserving the healthy tissue of the uterus. This surgery is ideal for women who wish to have children or retain their uterus for other reasons. However, new fibroids can develop, and all surgical risks apply.

Hysterectomy

Hysterectomy involves removing the uterus and is the only definitive cure for fibroids. It is often performed when fibroids are large, cause heavy bleeding, or the woman is near or past menopause and does not want children. Hysterectomy can be done through the abdomen, vagina, or laparoscope. While generally safe, hysterectomy is a major surgery with significant risks and requires several weeks for recovery.

Endometrial Ablation

This procedure removes or destroys the lining of the uterus to control heavy bleeding. It is usually a minor procedure with quick recovery but prevents future pregnancies.

Myolysis

Myolysis involves inserting a needle into the fibroids and using electric current or freezing to destroy them, typically guided by laparoscopy.

Uterine Fibroid Embolization

The uterine fibroid embolization (UFE) procedure involves threading a thin tube into the blood vessels supplying the fibroid and injecting particles to block blood flow, causing the fibroid to shrink. UFE is suitable for women who have heavy bleeding, pain, or pressure from fibroids and who do not wish to have a hysterectomy or children in the future. While complications are rare, early menopause can occur, and more long-term research is needed to determine the recurrence rate of fibroids after UFE.

NEW TREATMENTS FOR UTERINE FIBROIDS

Some emerging treatments are not yet standard, and insurance coverage may vary:

- **Radiofrequency ablation.** It uses heat to destroy fibroid tissue without harming surrounding uterine tissue. The fibroids shrink in size, with most women returning to normal activities within a few days.
- **Anti-hormonal drugs.** They may provide symptom relief without bone-thinning side effects.[1]

[1] Office on Women's Health (OWH), "Uterine Fibroids," U.S. Department of Health and Human Services (HHS), February 19, 2021. Available online. URL: www.womenshealth.gov/a-z-topics/uterine-fibroids. Accessed July 15, 2024.

Section 23.4 | Female Sterilization Methods and Their Effectiveness

Laparoscopic, abdominal, and hysteroscopic methods of female sterilization are available in the United States. These procedures can often be performed in an outpatient setting. Fewer than 1 out of 100 women become pregnant in the first year after female sterilization. Because these methods are intended to be irreversible, women should be counseled about the permanency of sterilization and the availability of long-acting, reversible contraception. Female sterilization does not protect against sexually transmitted diseases (STDs); consistent and correct use of male latex condoms reduces the risk of STDs, including human immunodeficiency virus (HIV).

HYSTEROSCOPIC STERILIZATION

Reliability for Contraception

Before relying on hysteroscopic sterilization for contraception, a hysterosalpingogram (HSG) must be performed three months after the procedure to confirm bilateral tubal occlusion. Women should abstain from sexual intercourse or use additional contraceptive protection until bilateral tubal occlusion is confirmed.

LAPAROSCOPIC AND ABDOMINAL STERILIZATION

Reliability for Contraception

Women can rely on sterilization for contraception immediately after laparoscopic and abdominal procedures, with no additional contraceptive protection needed.

COMMENTS AND EVIDENCE SUMMARY

HSG confirmation is necessary to confirm bilateral tubal occlusion after hysteroscopic sterilization. The inserts used in hysteroscopic sterilization in the United States are placed into the fallopian tubes and require three months for adequate fibrosis and scarring, leading to bilateral tubal occlusion. During this period, effective contraception should be used. If compliance is a concern, a DMPA injection may be considered at the time of sterilization to ensure contraception for three months. Unlike laparoscopic and abdominal sterilizations, the pregnancy risk beyond seven years has not been studied for hysteroscopic sterilization.

Long-Term Effectiveness

Pregnancy risk with at least 10 years of follow-up has been studied among women who underwent laparoscopic and abdominal sterilizations. Although these methods are highly effective, pregnancies can still occur many years after the procedure, especially among younger women.

Systematic Review of Hysteroscopic Sterilization

A systematic review identified 24 studies reporting on pregnancies after hysteroscopic sterilization. Few pregnancies occurred among women with confirmed bilateral tubal occlusion; however, few studies included long-term follow-up beyond seven years. Most pregnancies after hysteroscopic sterilization occurred in women without confirmed bilateral tubal occlusion at three months due to lack of follow-up or misinterpretation of HSG results. Some pregnancies occurred within three months of placement among women who were already pregnant at the time of the procedure, did not use alternative contraception, or experienced failures of alternative contraception. Most pregnancies occurred due to deviations from U.S. Food and Drug Administration (FDA) directions, which include placement in the early follicular phase, imaging at three months to document proper placement, and using effective alternative contraception until documented occlusion.

LEVEL OF EVIDENCE

- **Level II-3 (Fair, Direct)**. The evidence from studies on hysteroscopic sterilization, highlighting the importance of following FDA guidelines to minimize the risk of pregnancy.[1]

[1] "Female Sterilization," Centers for Disease Control and Prevention (CDC), March 27, 2023. Available online. URL: www.cdc.gov/reproductivehealth/contraception/mmwr/spr/female_sterilization.html. Accessed July 8, 2024.

Section 23.5 | **Endometrial Ablation**

WHAT IS ENDOMETRIAL ABLATION?

Endometrial ablation is a minimally invasive surgical procedure used to treat heavy menstrual bleeding by destroying the endometrial tissue, which lines the uterus. This procedure aims to reduce menstrual bleeding to normal or lighter levels.

CANDIDATES FOR ENDOMETRIAL ABLATION

Endometrial ablation is recommended for premenopausal patients with heavy menstrual bleeding due to benign (non-cancerous) causes who have completed childbearing. You are NOT a candidate if you:

- are pregnant or wish to become pregnant in the future
- have had a previous endometrial ablation or resection
- are on medications that thin the uterine muscles (e.g., long-term steroid use)
- have an intrauterine device (IUD) in place
- have abnormal vaginal bleeding that has not been evaluated
- have a known or suspected abdominal, pelvic, or gynecological cancer
- have conditions that weaken the uterine muscle layer
- have an active genital, pelvic, or urinary tract infection

HOW IS ENDOMETRIAL ABLATION PERFORMED?

Endometrial ablation is typically performed as an outpatient procedure. During the procedure, your health-care provider may need to dilate your cervix to insert the ablation device. Energy is then delivered to destroy the uterine lining, and the handpiece is removed afterward.

ENDOMETRIAL ABLATION DEVICES

The U.S. Food and Drug Administration (FDA) has approved various endometrial ablation devices that use different methods to destroy the endometrial tissue, including:

- heated gas
- radiofrequency energy
- heated saline
- microwave energy
- heated fluid within a balloon
- heated water vapor
- extreme cold (cryotherapy) using nitrous oxide within a balloon

WHAT TO KNOW BEFORE UNDERGOING ENDOMETRIAL ABLATION

Discuss the procedure with your health-care provider, including where and how it will be performed and the type of anesthesia used. You will need someone to drive you home after the procedure. Post-procedure, you will be evaluated for your readiness to go home and given follow-up instructions.

BENEFITS, COMMON SIDE EFFECTS, AND RISKS

Benefits

- reduction in menstrual bleeding
- improvement in quality of life (QOL)

Common Side Effects

- pain and cramping
- nausea
- vaginal discharge, bleeding, or spotting
- temporary diarrhea or headache

Risks (Immediate)

- deep injury to the uterus (perforation or burns)
- injury to abdominal organs (bowel or bladder)
- vaginal, vulvar, or skin burns
- infection
- hemorrhage
- air or gas embolism
- need for additional surgery (including possible hysterectomy)

Risks (Long Term)

- new menstrual pain (especially in patients with prior tubal ligation)
- collection and retention of blood in the uterus due to cervical narrowing
- difficulty diagnosing endometrial cancer due to scarring
- return of heavy menstrual bleeding, possibly requiring further treatment

IMPORTANT CONSIDERATIONS

Pregnancies following endometrial ablation can be dangerous. To avoid pregnancy, permanent sterilization or reversible contraception until menopause is necessary. Endometrial ablation does not protect against future pregnancy.

DISCUSS WITH YOUR HEALTH-CARE PROVIDER

If considering endometrial ablation, discuss:

- any problems you may have
- treatment options and whether you are a candidate
- the type of endometrial ablation device used, and its risks and benefits
- what to expect post-procedure and when to contact your provider with any problems

Ensure you receive patient labeling for the endometrial ablation device for more detailed information.[1]

Section 23.6 | Pelvic Organ Prolapse Repair

WHAT IS PELVIC ORGAN PROLAPSE?

Pelvic organ prolapse (POP) occurs when the tissue and muscles of the pelvic floor can no longer support the pelvic organs, causing

[1] "Endometrial Ablation for Heavy Menstrual Bleeding," U.S. Food and Drug Administration (FDA), October 25, 2021. Available online. URL: www.fda.gov/medical-devices/surgery-devices/endometrial-ablation-heavy-menstrual-bleeding. Accessed July 8, 2024.

them to drop from their normal position. The pelvic organs include the vagina, cervix, uterus, bladder, urethra, and rectum. The bladder is the most commonly involved organ in POP.

CAUSES AND RISK FACTORS

Supporting muscles and tissue of the pelvic floor may become torn or stretched due to:

- labor or childbirth
- age-related weakening
- genetic predisposition
- connective tissue disorders
- obesity
- frequent constipation

SYMPTOMS

Many women have some degree of POP, but not all experience symptoms. When symptoms do occur, they may include:

- pelvic discomfort or pain
- pressure in the pelvic area
- bulge of tissue or organs protruding to or past the vaginal opening
- urinary incontinence
- sexual difficulties

DIAGNOSIS

Consulting with a health-care provider is crucial for the proper diagnosis of POP.

TREATMENT OPTIONS FOR PELVIC ORGAN PROLAPSE

Nonsurgical Treatment Options

- **Pelvic floor exercises**. Strengthen the pelvic floor by contracting and relaxing the muscles around the urethra, vagina, and rectum. Commonly referred to as "Kegels."
- **Pessary**. A removable device inserted into the vagina to support the prolapsed pelvic organ(s).

Surgical Treatment Options

Surgery is not necessary for all women with POP. It may be recommended for those with significant discomfort or pain affecting their quality of life (QOL). Factors to consider include:

- the specific organ(s) that have prolapsed
- severity of prolapse
- desire for future children
- age
- sexual activity
- severity of symptoms

Surgical options include:

- restoring the normal position of the vagina
- repairing tissue around the vagina
- permanently closing the vaginal canal, with or without removing the uterus (colpocleisis)

Some women with POP may also experience urinary incontinence. During surgery, a procedure to prevent or decrease urine leakage, which may involve surgical mesh, might be performed.

WHAT SHOULD YOU DO IF SURGICAL MESH WAS USED TO REPAIR YOUR PELVIC ORGAN PROLAPSE TRANSVAGINALLY?

1. **Routine check-ups.** Continue with annual and routine follow-up care.
2. **Notify health-care provider.** Report any complications or symptoms such as persistent vaginal bleeding, discharge, pelvic or groin pain, or pain during sexual intercourse.
3. **Inform about mesh use.** Let your health-care provider know you have surgical mesh, especially if you plan to have another surgery or medical procedure.
4. **Discuss questions.** Talk to your health-care provider about any concerns or questions.
5. **Report problems.** Submit a voluntary report about any problems experienced with surgical mesh for POP repair through MedWatch, the FDA Safety Information

and Adverse Event Reporting program's website (www.accessdata.fda.gov/scripts/medwatch/index.cfm).

6. **Confirm mesh use**. If you had transvaginal POP surgery but are unsure whether mesh was used, ask your surgeon at your next visit.[1]

[1] "Pelvic Organ Prolapse (POP)," U.S. Food and Drug Administration (FDA), April 16, 2024. Available online. URL: www.fda.gov/medical-devices/urogynecologic-surgical-mesh-implants/pelvic-organ-prolapse-pop. Accessed July 15, 2024.

Chapter 24 | **Urological Surgeries**

Chapter Contents

Section 24.1 | **Circumcision**

WHAT IS CIRCUMCISION?

Circumcision is the removal of the foreskin, the skin that covers the tip of the penis. It is a decision often made before a new baby leaves the hospital. The American Academy of Pediatrics (AAP) does not recommend routine circumcision because the medical benefits do not outweigh the risks. However, parents should also consider their religious, cultural, and personal preferences when deciding whether to circumcise their son.

BENEFITS AND RISKS OF CIRCUMCISION

Possible Benefits

- **Lower risk of urinary tract infections (UTIs).** UTIs affect only 1 percent or less of men who are not circumcised.
- **Lower risk of penile cancer.** Penile cancer is very rare in both circumcised and uncircumcised men.
- **Possible lower risk of sexually transmitted infections (STIs).** Practicing safe sex, including using a condom, is the best protection against STIs.[1]

Additional Health Benefits

- **Human immunodeficiency virus (HIV) reduction.** Circumcision can reduce a male's chances of acquiring HIV by 50 to 60 percent during heterosexual contact with female partners with HIV.
- **Reduced risk of other infections.** Circumcised men have lower risks of syphilis (by 42%), genital ulcer disease (by 48%), genital herpes (by 28 to 45%), and high-risk strains of human papillomavirus (by 24 to 47%).
- **Partner benefits.** Circumcision does not reduce the chances of HIV transmission to female partners but does

[1] Office on Women's Health (OWH), "Circumcision," U.S. Department of Health and Human Services (HHS), February 22, 2021. Available online. URL: www.womenshealth.gov/pregnancy/getting-ready-baby/circumcision. Accessed July 15, 2024.

reduce the chance of a female partner acquiring a new syphilis infection by 59 percent. It also lowers the risk of cervical cancer in female sexual partners and infant urinary tract infections in male infants.[2]

Risks

- **Pain**. Numbing medicine can be applied to the baby's penis to lessen pain.
- **Bleeding or infection**. There is a low risk of bleeding or infection.[3]

CONSIDERATIONS DURING THE DECISION-MAKING PROCESS

Health Benefits

- Circumcision can reduce the risk of acquiring HIV, syphilis, genital ulcer disease, genital herpes, and high-risk strains of human papillomavirus associated with cancer.
- Observational studies suggest circumcision lowers the risk of penile cancer, cervical cancer in female sexual partners, and infant UTIs.

Health Risks

- The overall risk of adverse events associated with male circumcision is low.
- Minor bleeding and inflammation are the most common complications.
- The rate of adverse events for medically attended male circumcision is 0.4 percent for infants under one year, about 9 percent for children ages 1–9 years, and about 5 percent for males 10 years and older.
- Severe complications are exceedingly rare.
- Adult men who undergo circumcision generally report minimal or no change in sexual satisfaction or function.

[2] "Male Circumcision for HIV Prevention," Centers for Disease Control and Prevention (CDC), March 6, 2024. Available online. URL: www.cdc.gov/nchhstp-newsroom/factsheets/male-circumcision-for-hiv-prevention.html. Accessed July 15, 2024.
[3] See footnote [1].

Stage of Life

- Circumcision is simpler, safer, and less expensive for newborns and infants than for adult males.
- Delaying circumcision until adolescence or adulthood allows the male to participate in or make the decision but may diminish potential sexual health benefits and increase risks.

INFORMED CHOICE

Circumcision is a voluntary procedure. The decision should be made in consultation with a health-care provider, considering personal, cultural, religious, and ethical beliefs.[4]

Section 24.2 | Prostate Cancer Surgery

WHAT IS PROSTATE CANCER?

Prostate cancer is a disease where malignant (cancer) cells form in the tissues of the prostate, a gland in the male reproductive system. The prostate is located just below the bladder and in front of the rectum, surrounding part of the urethra. It is about the size of a walnut and produces fluid that is part of semen.

PREVALENCE

Prostate cancer is most common in older men. In the United States, about one in eight men will be diagnosed with prostate cancer.

SIGNS OF PROSTATE CANCER

Prostate cancer may cause symptoms such as:

- trouble starting the flow of urine
- frequent urination, especially at night

[4] See footnote [2].

- trouble emptying the bladder completely
- weak or interrupted flow of urine

Advanced stages of prostate cancer may present with:
- persistent pain in the back, hips, or pelvis
- symptoms of anemia such as shortness of breath, fatigue, rapid heartbeat, dizziness, or pale skin

Other conditions, such as benign prostatic hyperplasia (BPH), can cause similar symptoms.

DIAGNOSING PROSTATE CANCER

A transrectal biopsy is used to diagnose prostate cancer and determine the grade (Gleason score). This involves removing tissue from the prostate with a needle inserted through the rectum, guided by ultrasound or MRI.

- **Pathologist analysis**. The tissue is examined under a microscope to detect cancer cells.
- **Gleason score**. The grade of the cancer cells ranges from 6 to 10. Higher scores indicate more aggressive cancer:
  - 6: Low-grade cancer.
  - 7: Medium-grade cancer.
  - 8–10: High-grade cancer.

TREATMENT OPTIONS FOR PROSTATE CANCER

Surgery

Patients with tumors confined to the prostate gland may undergo surgery. The types of surgery include:

- **Radical prostatectomy (RP)**. Removal of the prostate, surrounding tissue, and seminal vesicles. Types of RP include:
  - **Open radical prostatectomy**. An incision is made in the lower abdomen or perineum.
  - **Radical laparoscopic prostatectomy**. Several small incisions are made in the abdomen for laparoscopic instruments.

    - **Robot-assisted laparoscopic radical prostatectomy**. Similar to laparoscopic surgery but uses robotic arms controlled by the surgeon.
- **Pelvic lymphadenectomy (PLND)**. Removal of lymph nodes in the pelvis to check for cancer cells.
- **Transurethral resection of the prostate (TURP)**. Removal of prostate tissue using a resectoscope inserted through the urethra, primarily to relieve symptoms.

Potential Surgical Complications

- impotence
- urinary or fecal incontinence
- shortening of the penis
- inguinal (groin) hernia—bulging of fat or part of the small intestine through weak muscles into the groin

Cryosurgery

Cryosurgery, also known as "cryotherapy," uses freezing to destroy prostate cancer cells, guided by ultrasound. This treatment can cause impotence and incontinence.

Prostate cancer is a prevalent disease among older men, with various symptoms and treatment options. Early diagnosis and appropriate treatment can significantly affect the quality of life (QOL) and outcomes for patients. Discussing symptoms and treatment options with a health-care provider is crucial for managing prostate cancer effectively.[1]

Section 24.3 | **Urinary Incontinence Surgery**

UNDERSTANDING BLADDER CONTROL PROBLEMS

Bladder control problems significantly affect how a person manages or releases urine. One common issue is urinary incontinence (UI), the

[1] "Prostate Cancer Treatment (PDQ®)–Patient Version," National Cancer Institute (NCI), February 16, 2023. Available online. URL: www.cancer.gov/types/prostate/patient/prostate-treatment-pdq. Accessed April 26, 2024.

accidental loss or leaking of urine. UI is not a disease but a condition often related to other health issues, such as prostate problems or pregnancy.

Bladder control problems can range from minor annoyances to significant disruptions in quality of life (QOL). These problems can cause embarrassment or fear, leading to a reluctance to participate in activities. For instance, you might lose urine while running or coughing or leak before reaching a toilet.

Bladder control problems are common, and proper treatment can improve QOL. It is important to discuss urine leaks with a health-care professional, who can suggest simple lifestyle changes or treatments to manage symptoms. Health-care professionals, such as gynecologists, urologists, and geriatricians, are well-versed in discussing and treating these issues.

TYPES OF BLADDER CONTROL PROBLEMS

Bladder control problems are identified by their symptoms. The most common types include:

- **Stress incontinence**. Leakage occurs during movements like coughing, sneezing, laughing, or physical activity that puts pressure on the bladder.
- **Urgency incontinence**. A strong urge to urinate causes leaks before reaching the toilet. This is often referred to as "overactive bladder" and occurs when bladder muscles and nerves do not coordinate properly.
- **Reflex incontinence**. Urine leaks without warning or an urge to urinate, often due to nerve damage from conditions like multiple sclerosis (MS) or trauma such as a spinal cord injury (SCI).
- **Overflow incontinence**. The bladder does not empty completely, leading to leakage as the bladder becomes too full.
- **Functional incontinence**. Physical disabilities or cognitive issues prevent reaching the toilet in time, such as difficulty unbuttoning pants due to arthritis or not recognizing the need to urinate due to Alzheimer disease (AD).

- **Temporary incontinence**. Short-term incontinence caused by temporary situations like certain medications or illnesses such as urinary tract infections (UTIs).
- **Bedwetting (nocturnal enuresis)**. Occurs in both children and adults, often due to factors like medication, caffeine, alcohol consumption, or underlying health conditions such as diabetes insipidus or obstructive sleep apnea (OSA).

COMPLICATIONS OF BLADDER CONTROL PROBLEMS

Bladder control problems can lead to several complications, including:

- **Reduced physical activity**. Fear of leakage during activities may lead to decreased physical exercise, affecting overall health.
- **Emotional distress**. The lifestyle changes caused by bladder control problems can lead to depression or social anxiety.
- **Intimacy problems**. Concerns about leaking urine during sexual activity may affect intimacy.

RELATED BLADDER SYMPTOMS AND PROBLEMS

If you have UI, you are more likely to have other bladder symptoms or problems, such as:

- urinary frequency
- getting up from sleep to urinate, called "nocturia"
- difficulty urinating
- trouble emptying your bladder fully, called "urinary retention"
- dribbling urine after you think you have finished

When discussing other symptoms you may have with UI, health-care professionals may use the term lower urinary tract symptoms (LUTS).

Working with a health-care professional to prevent and treat these related symptoms and problems is important for the health of your bladder and your overall health.

TREATMENT FOR BLADDER CONTROL PROBLEMS

If lifestyle changes are not working for you, your health-care professional may prescribe medicine, a medical device, a bulking agent, or—as a last resort—surgery to help treat UI.

Medicines

Urgency incontinence may be treated with one of the following medicines as a pill, liquid, or patch to relax your bladder:

- anticholinergics
- beta-3 agonists
- tricyclic antidepressants (TCAs)

Health-care professionals may use botulinum toxin A, also known as "Botox," to treat UI when other medicines or self-care treatments do not work. Botox may be injected into the bladder. Injecting Botox into the bladder relaxes it, making more room for urine and lowering the chances of urine leaks.

In addition to anticholinergics, men with UI who have an enlarged prostate may also be prescribed:

- alpha-blockers
- 5-alpha reductase inhibitors
- phosphodiesterase-5 (PDE5) inhibitors

Medical Devices

- **Catheter**. Individuals with overflow incontinence may need to use a catheter to empty their bladder. Your health-care professional will teach you how to use a catheter. Proper hygiene is important for catheter use and to avoid a bladder infection.
- **Pessary**. Women may use a soft, plastic device called a "pessary," which is inserted into the vagina for stress incontinence. The pessary presses against the wall of your vagina and the nearby urethra. The pressure helps hold up the urethra, so you have less leaking. Another newer product to treat stress incontinence is a tampon-like disposable device that you can insert into your vagina for up to 12 hours at a time. The product

expands to push up against your urethra to help decrease leaks.

Bulking Agents

Gel or paste can be injected near your urinary sphincter to treat stress incontinence. The injected material bulks up the area around the urethra. The extra thickness helps close your bladder opening, so you leak less.

Electrical Nerve Stimulation

If medicines and lifestyle changes do not help your UI, your health-care professional may suggest electrical nerve stimulation for urgency incontinence and other symptoms. Electrical nerve stimulation changes your bladder's reflexes, using mild pulses of electricity to stimulate the nerves that control the bladder and sphincter muscles.

Surgery

- **Sling surgery**. The most common surgery to treat stress incontinence in women is the sling surgery. In sling surgery for women, a surgeon works through the vagina to insert a strip of material between the vagina and urethra. The surgeon may choose to use a synthetic mesh, a screen-like material that supports weakened or damaged tissue, or the surgeon may choose a biologic graft made from human or animal tissue. Although sling surgery with synthetic mesh can be successful and safe, complications can occur in some women. Your health-care professional can explain the risks and benefits of surgery for stress incontinence and what kind of results you can expect. Stress incontinence in men can be treated with the male sling—a procedure in which mesh is placed under the urethra, lifting and supporting the urethra and sphincter muscles.
- **Artificial urinary sphincter**. Stress incontinence in men can be treated by implanting an artificial urinary sphincter (AUS)—a device that helps keep the urethra closed to prevent leaks.

- **Surgery to remove a blockage**. Overflow incontinence caused by a blockage or a narrowed urethra can be treated with surgery to remove the blockage. Bladder outlet obstruction may occur in men who have an enlarged prostate. When other treatments do not work well enough, your health-care professional may suggest surgery, including minimally invasive surgery, to remove enlarged prostate tissue or to widen the urethra.
- **Bladder enlargement, or bladder augmentation**. If UI is caused by nerve damage, your health-care professional may suggest surgery to make your bladder larger. This procedure may allow your bladder to store more urine but can make it more difficult to empty, which may require you to use a catheter.

Health-care professionals can provide detailed information on the risks, benefits, and expected outcomes of each treatment option.[1]

Section 24.4 | **Urinary Diversion**

UNDERSTANDING URINARY DIVERSION

Urinary diversion is a surgical procedure that creates a new way for urine to exit the body when urine flow is blocked or when there is a need to bypass a diseased area in the urinary tract.

The urinary tract is the body's drainage system for removing urine, which is made of wastes and extra fluid. Normally, urine flows from the kidneys, through the ureters, to the bladder, and out the urethra. When urine cannot flow normally, it may build up in the bladder, ureters, or kidneys, causing pain, urinary tract infections (UTIs), urinary stones, damage to the urinary tract, or

[1] "Bladder Control Problems (Urinary Incontinence)," National Institute of Diabetes and Digestive and Kidney Diseases (NIDDK), July 2021. Available online. URL: www.niddk.nih.gov/health-information/urologic-diseases/bladder-control-problems. Accessed July 8, 2024.

kidney failure. If left untreated, a buildup of urine in the urinary tract can be life-threatening.

Urinary diversion may be temporary—rerouting urine flow for several days, weeks, or months until normal flow can resume—or permanent, creating a lasting change in how urine flows through the body.

REASONS FOR URINARY DIVERSION

The most common reason for a urinary diversion is bladder cancer, which requires the removal of the bladder, a procedure called a "cystectomy." Other reasons include:

- nerve damage to the bladder from birth defects like spina bifida, spinal cord injury (SCI), or multiple sclerosis (MS)
- chronic inflammation of the bladder from severe interstitial cystitis (IC), recurrent UTIs, or chronic urinary retention (CUR)
- conditions causing external pressure on the urethra or ureters
- CUR from an enlarged prostate or benign prostatic hyperplasia (BPH)
- permanent bladder damage from radiation therapy
- severe urinary incontinence (UI) not manageable with standard treatments
- trauma to the bladder, urethra, or pelvis
- tumors in the genitourinary tract or adjacent tissues and organs
- urinary stones

TYPES OF URINARY DIVERSIONS

Bladder Catheterization

Bladder catheterization involves inserting a thin, flexible tube (catheter) into the bladder to drain urine into a collection bag outside the body. The types of urinary catheters include:

- **Foley catheter**. Inserted into the bladder through the urethra.
- **Suprapubic catheter**. Inserted into the bladder through a small hole in the skin beneath the belly button.

Catheters may remain in place for several days or weeks after urinary tract surgery or blockage treatment and, in some cases, may be permanent. Long-term catheters need periodic replacement.

Cystostomy

A cystostomy is a surgical procedure in which a small tube is inserted into the bladder through the skin of the lower abdomen, allowing urine to drain into an external bag.

Nephrostomy

During a nephrostomy, a small tube (nephrostomy tube) is inserted through the back skin into the kidney, allowing urine to drain into an external bag (see Figure 24.1). This may be needed when treated for a kidney stone or if the ureters are blocked or inflamed.

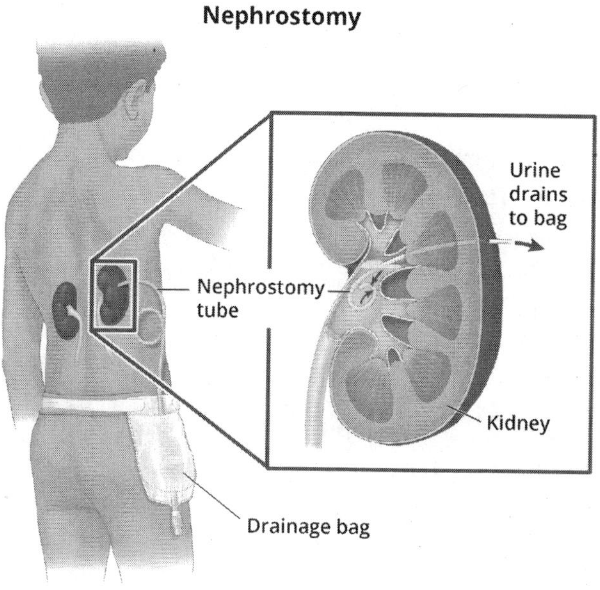

Figure 24.1. Nephrostomy

National Institute of Diabetes and Digestive and Kidney Diseases (NIDDK)

Ureteral Stent

A ureteral stent is a thin, flexible tube inserted into the ureter to help urine flow from the kidney to the bladder. It is usually temporary but can be used permanently to manage ureter blockages. Long-term stents need periodic replacement.

Urostomy

An urostomy is a stoma (opening) in the abdomen connected to the urinary tract that allows urine to drain freely. Urine is collected in an external pouch called a "urostomy pouch."

Types of urostomy include:

- **Ileal conduit**. A piece of the intestine creates a passageway for urine, which flows through the intestine piece and out of the stoma (see Figure 24.2).
- **Cutaneous ureterostomy**. One or both ureters are attached directly to a stoma in the abdomen (see Figure 24.3).

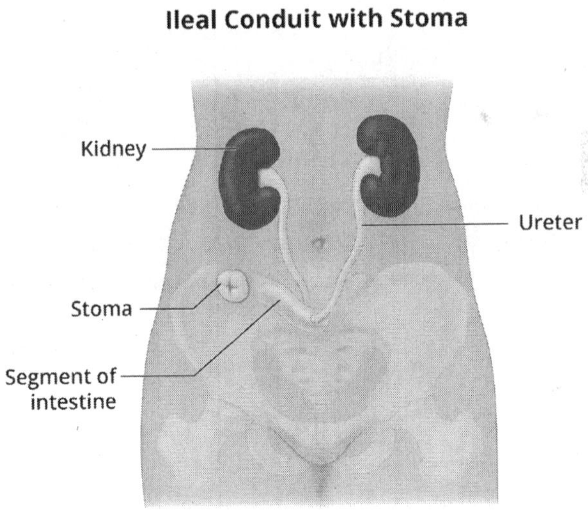

Figure 24.2. Ileal Conduit with Stoma

National Institute of Diabetes and Digestive and Kidney Diseases (NIDDK)

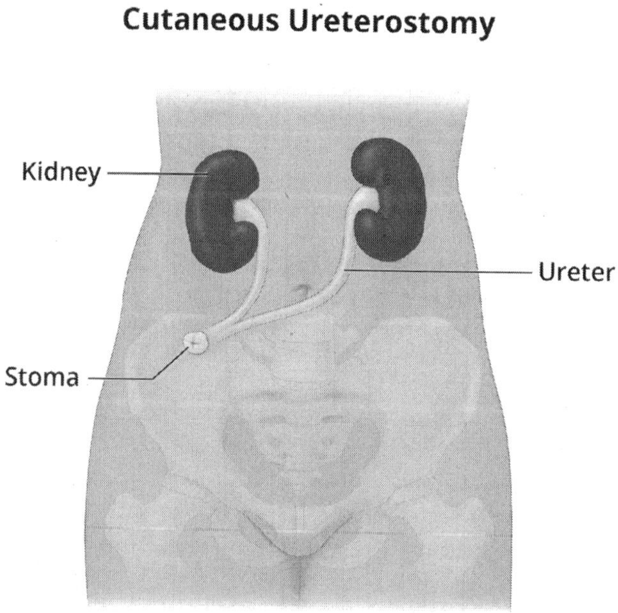

Figure 24.3. Cutaneous Ureterostomy

National Institute of Diabetes and Digestive and Kidney Diseases (NIDDK)

Continent Urinary Diversion

Continent urinary diversion collects and stores urine inside the body until it is drained using a catheter or urinated through the urethra.

Types include:

- **Continent cutaneous reservoir**. An internal pouch made from the bowel stores urine. Urine is drained by inserting a catheter into the stoma (see Figure 24.4).
- **Bladder substitute (neobladder)**. An internal reservoir made from the bowel holds urine. Urine flows through the ureters into the bladder substitute, and the individual urinates through the urethra.

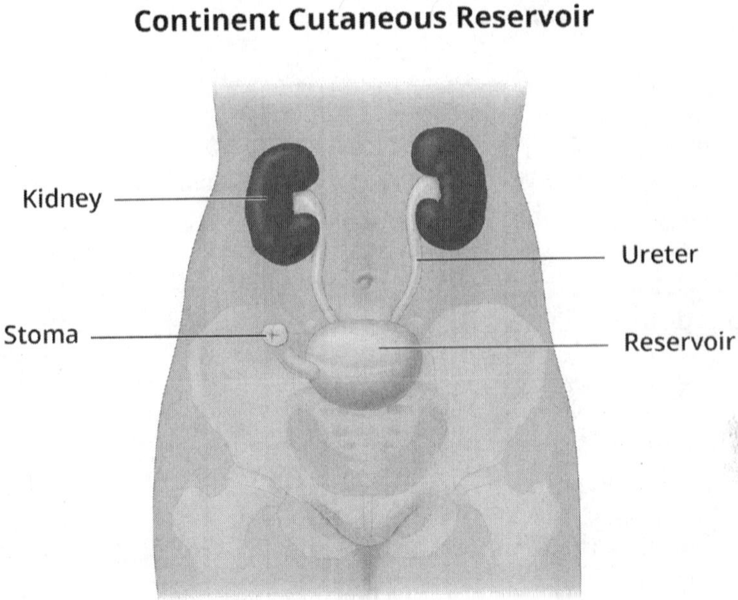

Figure 24.4. Continent Cutaneous Reservoir

National Institute of Diabetes and Digestive and Kidney Diseases (NIDDK)

POST-SURGERY EXPECTATIONS AND CARE

A nurse will teach you how to manage and care for your urinary diversion. Always wash your hands before and after care to prevent infection.

Caring for a Stoma

Daily care includes:

- gently wiping away mucus
- washing with warm water (using a mild soap if needed)
- thoroughly rinsing and drying
- avoiding products with oils, fragrance, deodorants, alcohol, or harsh chemicals
- inspecting for skin changes or irritation

Living with a Urostomy Pouch, Continent Cutaneous Reservoir, or Bladder Substitute

UROSTOMY POUCH

Care includes:

- emptying the pouch when one-third to one-half full
- changing the pouch one to two times per week
- keeping the skin around the stoma clean

Pouches are designed to prevent leaks, protect the skin, and avoid odor.

CONTINENT CUTANEOUS RESERVOIR

Care includes:

- emptying the pouch every two hours initially, then every four to six hours
- cleaning the skin around the stoma before and after catheter use
- flushing the internal pouch periodically

BLADDER SUBSTITUTE (NEOBLADDER)

Care includes:

- emptying the neobladder every two to three hours initially, then every four to six hours
- using a catheter if necessary
- flushing the neobladder periodically to remove mucus

INFECTION PREVENTION

Prevent infection by drinking plenty of fluids and being vigilant for symptoms like fever, chills, nausea, and painful urination. Contact a health-care professional if you notice signs of infection.

ACTIVITIES AND RELATIONSHIPS

After healing, most people can return to their usual activities. However, if you engage in strenuous activities or contact sports, consult with a health-care professional.

Discuss any concerns about relationships and intimacy with a health-care professional. It is important to communicate openly with your partner about intimacy.

DIET

Most people can return to a normal diet. Some may need to avoid foods that cause strong-smelling urine. People with certain diversions may need vitamin B_{12} injections. Discuss dietary needs with your health-care professional.[1]

Section 24.5 | **Vasectomy (Male Sterilization)**

WHAT IS A VASECTOMY?

A vasectomy is a surgical procedure for male birth control. It involves cutting the vas deferens to block the tubes that carry sperm from the testicles. With a successful vasectomy, a man can no longer get a woman pregnant.

Sperm is produced in the testicles, stored in the epididymis, and travels through the vas deferens during ejaculation, mixing with seminal fluid to form semen. After a vasectomy, sperm is no longer present in the semen. Over time, the testicles produce less sperm, and the body harmlessly absorbs any remaining sperm.

HOW IS A VASECTOMY DONE?

A vasectomy is usually performed in a urologist's office. In some cases, it may be done in an outpatient surgery center or hospital due to patient anxiety or additional procedures.

Conventional Method

- **Incisions.** One or two small cuts are made in the scrotum.

[1] "Urinary Diversion," National Institute of Diabetes and Digestive and Kidney Diseases (NIDDK), June 2020. Available online. URL: www.niddk.nih.gov/health-information/urologic-diseases/urinary-diversion. Accessed April 26, 2024.

- **Access**. The vas deferens is accessed, a section is cut out, and the ends are cauterized or tied.
- **Closure**. The procedure is repeated on the other testicle, and the incisions are closed with stitches or skin glue.

No-Scalpel Method

- **Puncture hole**. A small puncture hole is made on one side of the scrotum.
- **Access**. The vas deferens is pulled through the hole, cut, and a section is removed. The ends are cauterized or tied.
- **Closure**. The procedure is repeated on the other testicle. No stitches are needed due to the small size of the puncture holes.

Most men go home the same day and fully recover within a week.

WHAT ARE THE RISKS OF VASECTOMY?

Although vasectomy is safe and effective, men should be aware of potential problems post-surgery and over time.

Surgical Risks

- **Discomfort, bruising, and swelling**. These usually resolve within two weeks.
- **Hematoma**. Bleeding under the skin causing painful swelling.
- **Infection**. Signs include fever, scrotal redness, and tenderness.

Other Risks

- **Granuloma**. A lump in the scrotum formed from leaked sperm.
- **Postvasectomy pain syndrome (PVPS)**. Pain occurring in some men post-vasectomy.
- **Vasectomy failure**. There is a small risk of failure, leading to unintended pregnancy. Among 1,000 vasectomies, 11 may

fail over two years, with half of these failures occurring within the first three months. Factors influencing failure include surgical techniques and the rare possibility of the vas deferens growing back together.

Risk of Regret

Vasectomy is a good choice for men or couples certain about not wanting more or any children. Most men and their spouses do not regret the decision. However, men who undergo vasectomy before age 30 are more likely to seek a vasectomy reversal in the future.[1]

[1] "Vasectomy," Eunice Kennedy Shriver National Institute of Child Health and Human Development (NICHD), February 18, 2022. Available online. URL: www.nichd.nih.gov/health/topics/vasectomy. Accessed July 8, 2024.

Chapter 25 | **Organ and Tissue Transplantation**

Chapter Contents

Section 25.1 | **Organ Allocation and Transplantation Processes**

HOW ORGAN ALLOCATION WORKS

In the United States, the demand for organs far exceeds the supply. To address this imbalance, organ allocation balances factors of justice and medical utility. Justice ensures fair consideration of candidates' circumstances and medical needs, while medical utility aims to increase the number of transplants performed and the length of time patients and organs survive.

THE MATCHING PROCESS

The computer system that matches donors and recipients first filters out transplant candidates who cannot match the donor. Factors include:

- blood type
- height or weight
- medical specifics related to the organ type (e.g., immune system matching for kidney or pancreas)

The system then prioritizes candidates based on national policies for each matching factor.

GEOGRAPHY'S ROLE

Due to the limited time organs can be preserved, candidates closer to the donor hospital are given priority.

THE RIGHT-SIZED ORGAN

Matching organ size is crucial for a successful transplant. For example, children often respond better to child-sized organs, and they are generally given first consideration for other children's organs.

FACTORS IN ORGAN ALLOCATION

Kidney

- waiting time
- level of donor/recipient immune system match

- pediatric status
- prior living donor
- distance from the donor hospital
- survival benefit

Heart

- medical urgency
- distance from the donor hospital

Lung

- survival benefit
- medical urgency
- waiting time
- distance from the donor hospital

Liver

- medical urgency
- distance from the donor hospital

PRESERVING ORGANS

Organs can only be preserved for a short time between removal from the donor and transplant into a recipient. They cannot be frozen and stored for days or weeks. Preservation times are:

- **Kidneys.** Usually transplanted within 36 hours.
- **Liver, pancreas, and intestines.** Typically transplanted within 12 hours.
- **Hearts and lungs.** Usually transplanted within six hours.

Transplant teams prefer the shortest possible preservation time to ensure a successful transplant, though commonly accepted ranges exist based on the organ type.[1]

[1] "How Organ Allocation Works," Health Resources and Services Administration (HRSA), September 23, 2014. Available online. URL: https://optn.transplant.hrsa.gov/patients/about-transplantation/how-organ-allocation-works. Accessed July 8, 2024.

TRANSPLANT PROCESS

Transplant data show increasing numbers of people receiving transplants annually, with many living longer after their transplants.

WAITING TIMES

Waiting times vary widely due to multiple factors, including:

- blood type
- tissue type
- height and/or weight of the transplant candidate
- size of the donated organ
- medical urgency
- time on the waiting list
- number of donors in the local area
- types of organ offers the transplant hospital will accept

Each patient's need is different, and these factors influence how long a patient waits for a transplant.

PATIENT NOTIFICATION

Patients often contact the Organ Procurement and Transplantation Network (OPTN) to check if they are on the national transplant waiting list. However, only the transplant hospital can provide this information. Patients should discuss their status with their transplant team.

The transplant program must inform patients in writing within 10 business days of registration on the national transplant waiting list, including the listing date. If a patient is not placed on the waiting list, the program must notify them in writing within 10 days after completing the evaluation. If the transplant team removes a patient from the list for any reason other than transplant or death, the program must inform the patient in writing within 10 business days.

This policy aims to improve communication between transplant centers and their patients and to help patients understand the listing and transplant process.

OPTIONS TO CONSIDER

Multiple Listing

Patients can be listed at hospitals in different parts of the country. Each hospital has its own rules regarding multiple listings. Being listed in more than one area does not guarantee a faster organ match, but it can increase the chances of receiving an organ offer.

Transferring Waiting Time

Patients can transfer their listings to a different transplant hospital, adding the waiting time from the original center to the time at the new hospital. This requires cooperation between the transplant teams at each hospital and notification to the OPTN.

Living Donation

In addition to deceased organ donation, patients may receive organs from living donors. Living donor kidney transplants are most common, but a living donor can also provide a segment of the liver, lung, pancreas, or intestine. Living donation offers more people the chance to receive transplants, often sooner than they would from a deceased donor.[2]

Section 25.2 | Kidney Transplantation

Some people with kidney failure may be able to have a kidney transplant. During transplant surgery, a healthy kidney from a donor is placed into your body. The new, donated kidney does the work your two kidneys used to do.

A kidney can be donated by someone you do not know who has recently died (a deceased donor) or from a living person—a relative, spouse, or friend. Due to the shortage of kidneys, patients on the waiting list for a deceased donor kidney may wait many years.

[2] "Transplant Process," Health Resources and Services Administration (HRSA), September 23, 2014. Available online. URL: https://optn.transplant.hrsa.gov/patients/about-transplantation/transplant-process. Accessed July 8, 2024.

A kidney transplant is a treatment for kidney failure; it is not a cure. You will need to take medicines every day to make sure your immune system does not reject the new kidney. You will also need to see your health-care provider regularly.

A working transplanted kidney does a better job of filtering wastes and keeping you healthy than dialysis. However, a kidney transplant is not for everyone. Your doctor may tell you that you are not healthy enough for transplant surgery.

PROCESS FOR GETTING A KIDNEY TRANSPLANT

If you want a kidney transplant, the process includes these steps:

1. **Tell your doctor or nurse you want to have a kidney transplant.**
2. **Referral to a transplant center**. Your doctor will refer you to a transplant center for tests to see if you are healthy enough to receive a transplant. Living donors need to be tested to make sure they are healthy enough to donate a kidney.
3. **Waiting list**. If you do not have a living donor, you will be placed on a waiting list to receive a kidney. You will have monthly blood tests while you wait for a kidney.
4. **Hospital admission**. You must go to the hospital to have your transplant as soon as you learn a kidney is available. If you have a living donor, you can schedule the transplant in advance.

Talk with Your Doctor

The first step is to talk with your doctor to find out whether you are a candidate for a transplant. If you are on dialysis, your dialysis team will also be part of the process. If you and your doctor think a kidney transplant is right, your doctor will refer you to a transplant center.

Get Tested at a Transplant Center

At the transplant center, you will meet members of your transplant team. You will have tests to make sure you are a good candidate for a transplant.

Tests will include blood tests and tests to check your heart and other organs to make sure you are healthy enough for surgery. Some conditions or illnesses could make a transplant less likely to succeed, such as cancer that is not in remission or current substance abuse.

You will also have tests to check your mental and emotional health. The transplant team must be sure you are prepared to care for a transplanted kidney. You will need to be able to understand and follow a schedule for taking the medicines you need after surgery.

In "cross-matching," the transplant team tests the donor's blood against your blood to help predict whether your body's immune system will accept or reject the new kidney.

If a family member or friend wants to donate a kidney and is a good match, she or he will need a health exam to make sure she or he is healthy enough to be a donor. If you have a living donor, you do not need to be on a waiting list for a kidney and can schedule the surgery when it is best for you, your donor, and your surgeon.

Testing and evaluation at the transplant center may take several visits over weeks to months.

Get on the Waiting List

If your tests show you can have a transplant, your transplant center will add your name to the waiting list. Wait times can range from a few months to years. Most transplant centers prefer people who have been on the waiting list the longest. Other factors, such as your age, where you live, and blood type, may make your wait longer or shorter.

A transplant center can place you on the waiting list for a donor's kidney if your kidney function is 20 percent or less—even if you are not on dialysis. While you wait for a kidney transplant, you may need to start dialysis.

Have Monthly Blood Tests

While you wait for a kidney, you will need monthly blood tests. The center must have a recent sample of your blood to match with any kidney that becomes available.

Have Your Kidney Transplant

During kidney transplant surgery, a surgeon places a healthy kidney into your body. You will receive general anesthesia before the surgery. The surgery usually takes three or four hours. Unless your damaged kidneys cause infections, high blood pressure (HBP), or are cancerous, they can stay in your body. Surgeons usually transplant a kidney into the lower abdomen near the groin.

If you are on a waiting list for a donor's kidney, you must go to the hospital to have your transplant surgery as soon as you learn that a kidney is available.

If a family member or friend is donating a kidney, you will schedule the surgery in advance. Your surgical team will operate on you and your donor at the same time, usually in side-by-side rooms. One surgeon will remove the kidney from the donor, while another prepares you to receive it.

TRANSPLANT TEAM MEMBERS

A successful transplant involves working closely with your transplant team. Members of the team include:

- **You**. You are an important part of your transplant team.
- **Your family members**. This may include your spouse, parents, children, or any other family member you would like to involve.
- **Transplant surgeon**. The doctor who places the kidney in your body.
- **Nephrologist**. A doctor specializing in kidney health may work closely with a nurse practitioner or a physician's assistant.
- **Transplant coordinator**. A specially trained nurse will be your point of contact, arrange your appointments, and teach you what to do before and after the transplant.
- **Pharmacist**. A person who tells you about all your medicines fills your prescriptions and helps you avoid unsafe medicine combinations and side effects.

- **Social worker**. A person trained to help you solve problems in your daily life and coordinate care needs after your transplant.
- **Dietitian**. An expert in food and nutrition who teaches you about the foods you should eat and avoid, and how to plan healthy meals.

Your transplant team will be able to provide the support and encouragement you need throughout the transplant process.

POST-TRANSPLANT RECOVERY

Many people feel much better right after having transplant surgery. For some people, it takes a few days for the new kidney to start working. You probably will need to stay in the hospital for several days to recover from surgery—longer if you have any problems after the transplant. You will have regular follow-up visits with your nephrologist after leaving the hospital.

If you have a living donor, the donor will probably stay in the hospital for several days. However, a new technique for removing a kidney for donation that uses a smaller cut may allow the donor to leave the hospital in two to three days.

Before you leave the hospital, you need to learn how to stay healthy and take care of your donor kidney. You will have to take one or more antirejection medicines—also called "immunosuppressants." Without medicine, your immune system may treat your donor kidney as foreign, or not your own, and attack your new kidney. Antirejection medicines may have side effects.

You may also need to take other medicines—for example, antibiotics to protect against infections. Your transplant team will teach you what each medicine is for and when to take each one. Be sure you understand the instructions for taking your medicines before you leave the hospital.

Monitoring Your New Kidney

Blood tests help you know your donor's kidney is working. Before you leave the hospital, you will schedule an appointment at the transplant center to test your blood. The tests show how well your kidneys are removing wastes from your blood.

At first, you will need regular checkups and blood tests at the transplant center or from your doctor. As time goes on, you will have fewer checkups.

Your blood tests may show that your kidney is not removing wastes from your blood as well as it should. You may also have other symptoms that your body is rejecting your donor's kidney. If you have these problems, your transplant surgeon or nephrologist may order a kidney biopsy.

POSSIBLE PROBLEMS AFTER A KIDNEY TRANSPLANT

The donated kidney may start working immediately or take up to a few weeks to make urine. If the new kidney does not start working immediately, you will need dialysis treatments to filter wastes and extra salt and fluid from your body until it starts working.

Other problems following a kidney transplant are similar to other pelvic surgeries and may include:

- bleeding
- infection, especially a bladder infection
- hernia
- pain or numbness along the inner thigh that usually goes away without treatment

Transplant rejection is rare right after surgery and can take days or weeks to occur. Rejection is less common when the new kidney is from a living donor than from a deceased donor.

Symptoms of Transplant Rejection

Transplant rejection often begins before you feel any changes. The routine blood tests that you have at the transplant center will reveal early signs of rejection. You may develop HBP or notice swelling because your kidney is not getting rid of extra salt and fluid in your body.

Your health-care provider will treat early signs of rejection by adjusting your medicines to help keep your body from rejecting your new kidney.

Transplant rejection is becoming less common. However, your body may reject the donor kidney, even if you do everything you should. If that happens, you may need to go on dialysis and go back on the waiting list for another kidney. Some people can get a second kidney transplant.

SEEK MEDICAL CARE RIGHT AWAY

When you are taking antirejection medicines, you are at a greater risk for infection. Antirejection medicines can dull symptoms of problems, such as infection. Call your transplant center right away if you are not feeling well or have:

- a fever of more than 100 °F
- drainage from your surgical scar
- burning when you pass urine
- a cold or cough that would not go away

Side Effects of Antirejection Medicines

Some antirejection medicines may change your appearance. Your face may get fuller, you may gain weight, or you may develop acne or facial hair. Not all people have these side effects.

Antirejection medicines weaken your immune system, which can lead to infections. In some people, over long periods, a weakened immune system can increase their risk of developing cancer. Some antirejection medicines cause cataracts, diabetes, extra stomach acid, HBP, and bone disease.

When used over time, these medicines may also cause liver or kidney damage in some people. Your transplant team will order regular tests to monitor the levels of antirejection medicines in your blood and to measure your liver and kidney function.

DIETARY CONSIDERATIONS WITH A KIDNEY TRANSPLANT

You have more choices about what to eat after you receive a kidney transplant than you would if you were on dialysis. However, you must work with a dietitian to develop an eating plan that can change in response to your medicines, test results, weight, and blood pressure.

PAYING FOR YOUR TRANSPLANT

The federal government health insurance program will pay for the transplant and care for three years after the transplant. Medicare will also pay for your donor's surgery and her or his care.

Paying for Medicines

Medicare and private insurance may help pay for your medicines. Additionally, drug companies give discounts to people who can show that they cannot afford to pay for their prescriptions. Talk with your transplant social worker to find out what resources may be available to help you pay for your transplant.[1]

Section 25.3 | Liver Transplantation

WHAT IS A LIVER TRANSPLANT?

A liver transplant is surgery to remove your diseased or injured liver and replace it with a healthy liver from another person, called a "donor." If your liver stops working properly, known as liver failure, a liver transplant can save your life.

WHEN DO PEOPLE NEED A LIVER TRANSPLANT?

People need a liver transplant when their liver fails due to disease or injury. For adults in the United States, the most common reasons for needing a liver transplant are:

- alcoholic liver disease
- cancers that start in the liver combined with cirrhosis

---

[1] "Kidney Transplant," National Institute of Diabetes and Digestive and Kidney Diseases (NIDDK), January 2018. Available online. URL: www.niddk.nih.gov/health-information/kidney-disease/kidney-failure/kidney-transplant. Accessed April 17, 2024.

- fatty liver disease (nonalcoholic steatohepatitis)
- cirrhosis caused by chronic hepatitis C

Biliary atresia is the most common reason children need a liver transplant. Doctors may also consider a liver transplant for rare disorders such as urea cycle disorders and familial hypercholesterolemia.

People may need a liver transplant due to acute liver failure, an uncommon condition most often caused by taking too much acetaminophen. Other causes include:

- adverse reactions to prescription medicines, illegal drugs, and herbal medicines
- viral hepatitis
- toxins
- blockage of the blood vessels to the liver
- autoimmune diseases
- genetic disorders

TYPES OF LIVER TRANSPLANT

Deceased Donor Transplants

Most livers for transplants come from people who have recently died, called "deceased donors." During a deceased donor transplant, surgeons remove your diseased or injured liver and replace it with the deceased donor's liver. Adults typically receive the entire liver from a deceased donor, though surgeons may split a liver into two parts, with the larger part going to an adult and the smaller part to a child or smaller adult.

Living Donor Transplants

In some cases, a healthy living person donates part of their liver, most often to a family member. This is known as a "living donor transplant." During this procedure, surgeons remove part of the living donor's healthy liver and replace it with your diseased or injured liver. Both the donor's and recipient's livers will grow back to normal size soon after the surgery. Living donor transplants are less common than deceased donor transplants.

LIVER TRANSPLANT PROCESS

Talk with Your Doctor about a Liver Transplant

The first step is to talk with your doctor to determine whether you are a candidate for a transplant. Doctors consider liver transplants only after ruling out all other treatment options. However, a liver transplant is not suitable for everyone. Your doctor may tell you that you are not healthy enough for surgery or have a medical condition that would make a transplant unlikely to succeed. If you and your doctor think a liver transplant is right, your doctor will refer you to a transplant center.

Visit a Transplant Center

During your first visit to a transplant center, health professionals will provide information about:

- the evaluation and approval process
- placement on the national waiting list
- reasons for being removed from the national waiting list
- the waiting period
- how people are selected for liver transplants
- surgery and recovery
- the long-term demands of living with a liver transplant, such as taking medicines for the rest of your life

Get Evaluated for a Liver Transplant

At the transplant center, you will undergo a series of evaluations and meet members of your transplant team. These evaluations may require several visits over weeks or months. Your transplant team may include:

- **Transplant coordinator**. A specially trained nurse who will be your point of contact, arrange appointments, and provide information before and after your transplant.
- **Transplant surgeons**. Specially trained doctors who perform the surgery and provide care before and after your transplant.

- **Hepatologist**. A doctor specializing in liver disease.
- **Insurance case manager**. A person who helps with your insurance coverage.
- **Financial coordinator**. A person who assists with financial matters.
- **Social worker**. A person who helps solve daily life problems and coordinate care needs.
- **Psychiatrist**. A doctor who assesses your mental and emotional readiness for caring for a new liver.
- **Dietitian**. An expert in food and nutrition.

Your team will ask about your medical history and perform medical tests, including:

- physical exam
- blood and urine tests
- imaging tests to view organs inside your body
- tests to check the function of your heart, lungs, and kidneys

The results of these tests will help determine:

- how likely you are to survive transplant surgery
- other diseases and conditions you may have
- the cause and severity of your liver disease

Your team will assess whether you are healthy enough for surgery. Some conditions or illnesses can make a liver transplant less likely to succeed. You may not be able to have a transplant if you have:

- a severe infection
- alcohol or drug abuse problems
- cancer outside the liver
- serious heart or lung disease

The transplant team will also evaluate whether you or your caregivers can understand and follow post-transplant care instructions and whether you have a strong support system. They will review your medical insurance and financial resources, as financial assistance programs may help with the cost of surgery, medicines, and care.

APPROVAL AND WAITING LIST

Get Approved for a Liver Transplant

The transplant center's selection committee will review your evaluation results. Each transplant center has its own guidelines, often posted on their websites, and follows national guidelines. Keep in mind that you may choose not to have a transplant even if approved.

Get Placed on the National Waiting List

If you are approved and do not have a living donor, the transplant center will place your name on the national waiting list for a liver from a deceased donor. If you have a living donor, the transplant center will not place you on the national waiting list.

The Organ Procurement and Transplantation Network (OPTN) and the United Network for Organ Sharing (UNOS) manage the national waiting list. Once you are added to the list, UNOS will notify you and your transplant center.

UNOS policies allow you to register with more than one transplant center to increase your chances of receiving a liver. Each center may require a separate medical evaluation.

Wait for a Match

The waiting period for a deceased donor transplant can range from less than 30 days to more than five years, depending on the urgency of your need and other factors such as age, location, blood type, body size, overall health, and the availability of a matching liver. UNOS policies prioritize those with the most urgent need to prevent death at the top of the list.

When a matching liver is found, your transplant team coordinator will contact you and ask you to come to the hospital immediately.

Confirm Living Donor Match

If a family member, spouse, or friend wants to be a living donor, the transplant team will ensure compatibility in blood types and body size. The potential donor will undergo medical tests and must be between 18 and 60 years old with an emotional tie to you.

PREPARING FOR LIVER TRANSPLANT SURGERY

How you prepare for surgery depends on the type of transplant:

- **Deceased donor transplant.** Your transplant team coordinator will call you as soon as a matching liver is found, and you must go to the hospital immediately.
- **Living donor transplant.** You will schedule your surgery four to six weeks in advance, and your transplant team coordinator will guide you and the donor on pre-surgery preparations.

LIVER TRANSPLANT SURGERY

Doctors will remove your diseased or injured liver and replace it with the donor's liver. The surgery can take up to 12 hours or longer and involves:

- general anesthesia
- intravenous (IV) and other lines for medicines and fluids
- monitoring of your heart and blood pressure

If you are receiving a liver from a deceased donor, your surgery will start when the liver arrives at the transplant center. If from a living donor, the surgical team will operate on you and the donor simultaneously.

POSSIBLE PROBLEMS OF LIVER TRANSPLANT SURGERY

Potential complications include:

- bleeding
- blood clots in your liver's blood vessels
- damage to the bile ducts
- failure of the donated liver
- infection
- rejection of the donated liver

POST-SURGERY CARE

After surgery, you will stay in the intensive care unit (ICU) for close monitoring and begin taking immunosuppressants to prevent organ rejection. Once stable, you will move to a regular hospital room.

The transplant team will educate you on self-care before discharge, including follow-up medical care, medication management, and recognizing potential problems.

GOING HOME AND RETURNING TO NORMAL ACTIVITIES

You can likely go home about two weeks after surgery while living donors can typically leave after one week. Most people return to normal activities, including work and physical activity, within a few months. Regular medical checkups will continue to ensure your liver functions properly. Women are often advised to wait at least a year after the transplant before getting pregnant.

ORGAN REJECTION

What Is Organ Rejection?

Organ rejection occurs when your immune system sees your transplanted liver as foreign and tries to destroy it. The highest risk period is within the first three to six months after the transplant.

Symptoms of Organ Rejection

Signs of rejection may include:

- abnormal liver blood test results
- fatigue
- abdominal pain or tenderness
- fever
- jaundice (yellowing of the skin and eyes)
- dark urine
- light-colored stools

Contact your doctor immediately if you experience symptoms of rejection. A liver biopsy may be performed to confirm rejection.

Preventing Organ Rejection

To prevent rejection, you must take immunosuppressants for the rest of your life. Rejection can occur if these medicines fail to control your immune response. In some cases, another transplant may be necessary.

SIDE EFFECTS OF IMMUNOSUPPRESSANTS

Immunosuppressants can cause side effects, including:

- increased susceptibility to infections
- brittle bones
- diabetes
- high blood pressure (HBP)
- high cholesterol and triglycerides
- kidney damage
- weight gain
- increased cancer risk

Inform your doctor about new medications, including over-the-counter (OTC) medicines, vitamins, and dietary supplements.

CARING FOR YOUR NEW LIVER

- Take medicines as prescribed.
- Consult your doctor before taking new medications.
- Keep medical appointments and scheduled blood draws.
- Avoid sick people.
- Report any illness to your doctor.
- Recognize symptoms of rejection and infection.
- Follow cancer screening recommendations.
- Stay up-to-date with vaccinations (avoid live vaccines).
- Discuss contraceptives and pregnancy risks with your doctor.

MAKING HEALTHY CHOICES

- Eat a balanced diet.
- Exercise regularly.

- Do not smoke.
- Avoid alcohol if you have a history of alcohol use disorder.
- Protect yourself from soil exposure and disease-transmitting organisms.

DIETARY CONSIDERATIONS AFTER A LIVER TRANSPLANT

What to Eat

Follow a healthy, well-balanced diet to aid recovery and maintain health. A dietitian can help create a suitable eating plan.

What to Avoid

Avoid grapefruit and grapefruit juice, as they can interfere with immunosuppressants. Also, avoid:

- water from lakes and rivers
- unpasteurized milk products
- raw or undercooked eggs, meats (especially pork and poultry), fish, and seafood

Limit intake of:

- salt
- cholesterol
- fat
- sugar[1]

Section 25.4 | **Heart Transplantation and Artificial Heart**

HEART TRANSPLANT

A heart transplant is surgery that removes a diseased heart and replaces it with a healthy heart from a deceased donor to improve your quality of life (QOL) and increase your lifespan. Heart

[1] "Liver Transplant," National Institute of Diabetes and Digestive and Kidney Diseases (NIDDK), March 2017. Available online. URL: www.niddk.nih.gov/health-information/liver-disease/liver-transplant. Accessed April 17, 2024.

transplant surgery is a kind of open-heart surgery performed in a hospital under anesthesia.

Recovery after Heart Transplant Surgery

After the surgery, you will recover in the hospital's intensive care unit (ICU) and stay in the hospital for up to three weeks. During your recovery, you may start a cardiac rehabilitation program. Before leaving the hospital, you will learn how to keep track of your overall health, monitor your weight, blood pressure, pulse, and temperature, and recognize the warning signs that your body may be rejecting your new heart. You will also learn to identify early signs of infection.

For the first three months after leaving the hospital, you will often return for tests to check for infection or rejection of your new heart, to see how well your heart is working, and to ensure you are recovering well. You can help prevent complications after a heart transplant by practicing good hygiene, getting routine vaccines and dental care, and making healthy lifestyle choices.

Risks of Heart Transplant

Heart transplant has some serious risks:

- **Primary graft dysfunction**. This happens when the donor heart fails and cannot function. This is the most common cause of death in the first month after a heart transplant.
- **Your immune system may reject your new heart**. Rejection is most likely to occur within six months after the transplant. You will need to take medicines for the rest of your life to suppress your immune system and help prevent your body from rejecting your new heart. These medicines weaken your immune system and increase your chance of infection. Their long-term use can also increase your risk of cancer, cause diabetes and osteoporosis, and damage your kidneys.
- **Cardiac allograft vasculopathy**. This is a common and serious complication of heart transplant. This aggressive type of atherosclerosis, or buildup of plaque

in the arteries, can block the heart's arteries over a few months or years and cause the donor heart to fail.
- **Over time, your new heart may fail due to the same reasons that caused your original heart to fail.** Some patients who have a heart transplant that fails may be eligible for another transplant.

Despite these risks, heart transplant has a good success rate. Survival rates are about 85 percent one year after surgery. Survival rates decrease by about 3–4 percent each additional year after surgery, mainly because of serious complications related to heart transplant.[1]

TOTAL ARTIFICIAL HEART

A total artificial heart (TAH) is a pump placed in the chest to replace damaged heart ventricles and valves. Ventricles are the chambers of the heart that pump blood to the lungs and other parts of the body.

Function and Structure

The TAH has ventricles made from polyurethane, a durable and flexible artificial material. Once the pump is placed in the chest, a machine called a "driver" controls the pump from outside the body. The pump and driver help blood flow to and from the heart, replacing the role of a healthy heart.

Your health-care provider will do tests and talk to you about what to expect during surgery. As with any surgery, TAH surgery can lead to serious problems such as blood clots or infection. During recovery, you may need to stay in the hospital to manage or prevent these problems. Before going home, health-care providers will help you learn how to protect and care for your TAH.

The TAH is mainly a temporary measure (often called a "bridge to transplant") to keep blood pumping while a person waits for a

[1] "Heart Treatments," National Heart, Lung, and Blood Institute (NHLBI), March 24, 2022. Available online. URL: www.nhlbi.nih.gov/health/heart-treatments-procedures. Accessed April 26, 2024.

donor's heart for a heart transplant. In the United States, only one TAH has been approved by the U.S. Food and Drug Administration (FDA), and it is only approved for use as a bridge to transplant. Scientists are still working to create a permanent artificial heart.

In some cases, people who are not candidates for a heart transplant may be able to receive a TAH through participation in a clinical trial.

How a Total Artificial Heart Works

The TAH replaces the lower chambers of the heart, called "ventricles." Tubes called "pneumatic drive lines" run through holes in the stomach area to connect the TAH pump to a machine outside the body called a "driver." The TAH then pumps blood through the major arteries to the lungs and the rest of the body.

The TAH has four mechanical valves that work like the heart's own valves to manage blood flow. These valves connect the TAH to the heart's upper chambers, called the "atria," and to the major arteries, including the pulmonary artery and the aorta. Once connected, the TAH acts like a healthy heart, allowing blood to flow normally.

The driver powers and controls the TAH. When used in the hospital, it is placed next to the bed. When outside the hospital, a portable driver that fits in a shoulder bag or backpack and weighs about 14 pounds is used. It can be recharged at home or in a car.

Who Needs a Total Artificial Heart?

The FDA approved the TAH as a bridge to a transplant. TAHs are used to keep people with heart failure alive while they wait for a heart transplant. TAHs have also been used for people living with other heart conditions as part of research into those conditions. Researchers are working on TAH devices that may be used as treatments for people who cannot have a transplant.

You may be a candidate for a TAH if you have advanced heart failure caused by the inability of your heart's ventricles to pump enough blood and if other treatments have not worked. You may also be a candidate if your body has rejected an earlier heart transplant.

A TAH may also be used for people with:

- an uncontrollable ventricular arrhythmia (VA)
- end-stage complications of congenital heart defects (CHD)
- ventricles that are not the right shape for a ventricular assist device (VAD)
- broken or ruptured ventricles
- a left ventricle that fails to work properly after a mechanical valve replacement surgery
- blood clots in the lining of the blood vessels and heart

Who Is Not Eligible for a Total Artificial Heart?

Your health-care provider will likely not recommend a TAH if you:

- are too small, although newer technologies are compact enough for smaller adults and some children
- may benefit instead from other treatments, including medicines
- have heart failure on only one side of your heart and could benefit from a heart treatment called a "VAD" instead
- cannot take anticlotting medicines, which are required as long as the TAH is in place

Preparing for Surgery

If you are not already in the hospital, you will probably spend at least a week there to get ready for TAH surgery. You will continue to take any heart medicines prescribed by your health-care provider.

You will meet with doctors specializing in the heart, including cardiologists and cardiac surgeons. You will get important information, such as how to prepare for your surgery and what to expect after. Ask your health-care provider to show you what the TAH device looks like and how it will be placed in your body.

Your providers will order tests to ensure your body is strong enough for surgery, including:

- **Blood tests**. To determine your blood type in case you need blood during surgery and to check how well your liver and kidneys work.

- **Chest imaging tests**. These tests take pictures of your heart, lungs, and the inside of your chest to ensure that the large TAH will fit.
- **Heart tests**. Include an electrocardiogram (ECG or EKG) to monitor your heart's rhythm and imaging tests to show how well blood moves through your heart and blood vessels.
- **Lung function tests**. To measure how well your lungs work and to help determine if you may need a ventilator after the surgery.

Some people receive extra nutrition through a feeding tube before receiving a TAH.

Surgery Overview

The surgery to connect the TAH is complicated and lasts five to nine hours.

SURGICAL TEAM

As many as 15 people may be in the operating room during the surgery:

- **Surgeons**. They perform the operation.
- **Surgical nurses**. They assist the surgeons.
- **Anesthesiologists**. They give you medicine to make you sleep during the surgery.
- **Specialists**. Also called "perfusionists," they oversee the heart-lung bypass machine, which keeps blood flowing through the body while the TAH is placed in the chest.
- **Engineers**. They assemble the TAH and ensure it is working well.

IMPLANTING THE TOTAL ARTIFICIAL HEART

Placing the TAH in your body and starting the heart pump is a multistep process:

- An anesthesiologist gives you medicine to make you sleep during the surgery and monitors your heart rate, blood pressure, oxygen levels, and breathing throughout the procedure.

- A breathing tube is placed in your windpipe through your mouth and connected to a ventilator machine to support your breathing during the surgery.
- The surgeon makes a cut into the chest bone and opens the sternum, a long, flat bone in the center of the chest.
- Medicines are administered to stop your heart so the surgeons can operate on it while it is not moving. A heart-lung bypass machine keeps oxygen-rich blood moving through your body during the surgery.
- The surgeon removes the heart's ventricles, attaches the TAH to the upper chambers of the heart, and connects it to the aorta and the pulmonary artery.
- After the TAH is attached, the surgical team turns off the heart-lung bypass machine and starts the TAH pump.
- The chest is usually left open for a day after surgery. If the TAH works properly and there is no unusual bleeding, the surgeon closes the chest.
- Once additional tests confirm that everything is working as it should, the chest is fully closed. Parts of the heart not removed are clearly marked, and the chest is closed in a way that can be reopened more easily when it is time for a heart transplant.

Post-Surgery Recovery

A hospital stay after TAH surgery may last a month or more. The recovery time depends on how healthy the person was before the surgery.

INITIAL RECOVERY

After surgery, you will first recover in the ICU. Your chest and abdomen may be sore or painful, and your health-care provider will give you medicines to manage the pain. A ventilator may still be needed to help with breathing. For a while, fluids and nutrition may be given through a feeding tube or an intravenous (IV) line in the arm. Health-care providers will monitor another IV line in the neck or leg to check how well the TAH works. A tube is also inserted into the urinary tract to drain urine and check kidney function.

MOVING TO A REGULAR HOSPITAL ROOM

A few days or more after surgery, you may be moved to a regular hospital room. Nurses experienced with TAHs and similar devices will manage your recovery. They help with sitting, getting out of bed, and walking around. Most people can get up and move around after two weeks. Nurses and physical therapists will assist with exercises to regain strength by gradually increasing activity.

Hospital staff will remove feeding, IV, and urine tubes as you strengthen. Eating regular food, going to the bathroom independently, and showering are signs of progress. This period is also used to teach you how to care for the TAH at home.

During hospital recovery, your family or friends can also learn how to care for the TAH to assist with your recovery at home.

Possible Surgery-Related Complications

Surgery to receive a TAH, like any surgery, carries some risks, including:

- **Blood clots**. Blood may clot more easily because it contacts the machine-made parts of the TAH. Clots can block blood vessels that deliver oxygen to vital organs, causing serious complications such as stroke, pulmonary embolism, or death. People with TAHs take anticlotting medicines for as long as they have the device.
- **Bleeding**. The surgery to connect a TAH is complex, and bleeding can occur in the chest during and after the surgery. Anticlotting medicine also increases the risk of bleeding by thinning the blood.
- **Infection**. After surgery, there is a higher risk of infection, so your health-care provider may give you medicine to lower this risk. You will be closely monitored for fever or other signs of infection.

- **Death**. During TAH surgery, as in any major surgery, there is a risk of death from the procedure or an adverse reaction to anesthesia medicines

Additional Risks and Complications

A TAH may prolong your life until a donor heart becomes available.

Between 60 and 80 percent of TAH recipients live long enough to receive a heart transplant. However, if they do not receive a heart transplant, less than 60 percent of people with a TAH survive for one year after surgery.

In addition to the risks of heart surgery, complications can arise after receiving a TAH, including:

- kidney infection and failure, which develop more often in people with a TAH than in those with ventricular assist devices
- QOL may be affected by the need for frequent changes and charging of the home-based driver. Hospital-based TAH drivers are also large and loud

Living with a Total Artificial Heart

Your recovery will continue after you leave the hospital. Over time, you must gradually increase your activity level, protect and care for your TAH, and exercise well.

After TAH surgery, you can do more activities than before. The driver that controls and powers the TAH is portable, allowing you to get out of bed, get dressed, and move around the house. It may even be possible to drive and engage in other activities outside. Talk to your health-care provider about the activity level that is safe for you.

Ongoing Care

You will need to see your provider regularly to monitor your recovery and take steps to prevent another heart problem.

SCHEDULE REGULAR CHECKUPS

Checkups with your provider or surgeon are essential to ongoing care after heart surgery. During these visits, you may have blood tests or heart tests such as EKG, echocardiography, or a stress test. These tests will show how your heart is working after surgery.

TAKE YOUR MEDICINE AS PRESCRIBED

As long as you have a TAH, you will need to take anticlotting medicine to prevent dangerous blood clots. Regular blood tests will help determine the correct dose. You will also need to take medicine to prevent infections. Your doctor may tell you how often to check your temperature to ensure you do not have a fever, a warning sign of infection.

MAKE HEART-HEALTHY LIFESTYLE CHANGES

Your provider may recommend lifestyle changes to help you stay healthy, including:

- choosing heart-healthy foods
- being physically active when it is safe to do so
- managing stress
- getting enough good-quality sleep

LEARN MORE ABOUT PROTECTING YOUR HEART

Your provider may refer you to cardiac rehabilitation, a medically supervised program for people recovering from heart problems. It usually includes exercise training, education on heart-healthy living, and counseling to reduce stress and help you recover. Your provider can help you find a cardiac rehabilitation program near your home.

Your health-care provider will also monitor you for complications that can develop after surgery, including:

- anemia
- high blood pressure (HBP)
- liver failure
- kidney failure[2]

---

[2] "What Is Total Artificial Heart?" National Heart, Lung, and Blood Institute (NHLBI), April 12, 2023. Available online. URL: www.nhlbi.nih.gov/health/total-artificial-heart. Accessed April 26, 2024.

Section 25.5 | **Lung Transplantation**

FUNCTION AND STRUCTURE OF THE LUNGS

The lungs are a pair of highly elastic and spongy organs in the chest. They are divided into lobes, with three on the right and two on the left. They are the main organs involved in breathing, taking in air, and providing a place for oxygen to enter the blood and for carbon dioxide to leave the blood.[1]

WHAT IS A LUNG TRANSPLANT?

A lung transplant is a surgery to remove a diseased lung and replace it with a healthy lung. Lung transplants are used to improve the quality of life (QOL) and extend the lifespan of people who have severe or advanced chronic lung conditions that do not respond to other treatments.[2]

TYPES OF LUNG TRANSPLANTS

Lung transplants may involve two lungs, a single lung, or a lobe of a lung. Transplants from deceased donors usually involve one or both whole lungs. In general, the most common diseases leading to a deceased donor lung transplant are:

- pulmonary fibrosis
- emphysema/chronic obstructive pulmonary disease (COPD)
- cystic fibrosis (CF)

Most lung lobe transplants, while rare, have been performed for patients with CF. The transplants can involve two living donors who each donate a lung lobe.[3]

[1] "Lung," Health Resources and Services Administration (HRSA), January 15, 2023. Available online. URL: https://optn.transplant.hrsa.gov/patients/by-organ/lung. Accessed April 26, 2024.
[2] "Lung Disease Treatments," National Heart, Lung, and Blood Institute (NHLBI), March 24, 2022. Available online. URL: www.nhlbi.nih.gov/health/lung-treatments. Accessed April 26, 2024.
[3] See footnote [1].

PROCEDURE FOR LUNG TRANSPLANT SURGERY

During a lung transplant, you will have general anesthesia and will not be awake for the surgery. A surgeon will:

- open your chest
- cut the main airway and blood vessels
- remove your diseased lung
- connect the healthy donor lung
- reconnect the blood vessels
- close your chest

After the surgery, you will recover in the hospital for one to three weeks. After leaving the hospital, you will visit your doctor often to ensure you are recovering well.

POST-SURGERY CARE

To help prevent your body from rejecting the new lung, you will need to take medicines for the rest of your life that suppress your immune system. Practicing good hygiene, getting annual vaccines, and adopting healthy lifestyle choices such as heart-healthy eating and not smoking are very important.

CONDITIONS LEADING TO LUNG TRANSPLANT

Lung transplants are used for:

- alpha-1 antitrypsin (AAT) deficiency
- chronic obstructive pulmonary disease (COPD)
- cystic fibrosis (CF)
- idiopathic pulmonary fibrosis (IPF)
- pulmonary hypertension
- sarcoidosis[4]

[4] See footnote [2].

Section 25.6 | **Pancreas and Islet Transplantation**

FUNCTION AND STRUCTURE OF THE PANCREAS

The pancreas is a gland located behind the stomach. It makes insulin, which controls the use of blood sugar throughout the body. It also makes enzymes that are used to digest food.

TYPES OF PANCREAS TRANSPLANTS

A pancreas transplant may involve either the whole pancreas or a pancreas segment. Whole organ transplants are far more common, but a segmental transplant is possible, especially if a living donor is involved. Many pancreas transplants also involve transplantation of the duodenum.

The kidney is frequently transplanted with the pancreas in the United States, as many people suffering from pancreas failure also have renal failure. In most cases, a kidney-pancreas transplant is performed from a deceased donor. However, some transplants have been performed using a living donor, with one kidney and a pancreas segment being donated.

REASONS FOR PANCREAS TRANSPLANTS

The reasons for pancreas transplants include:

- retransplant/graft failure
- type 1 diabetes
- type 2 diabetes
- diabetes secondary to chronic pancreatitis without pancreatectomy
- diabetes secondary to cystic fibrosis without pancreatectomy
- pancreatic cancer
- bile duct cancer
- other cancers
- pancreatectomy prior to pancreas transplant[1]

[1] "Pancreas," Health Resources and Services Administration (HRSA), February 2001. Available online. URL: https://optn.transplant.hrsa.gov/patients/by-organ/pancreas. Accessed April 17, 2024.

WHAT ARE ISLETS?

Pancreatic islets, also called "islets of Langerhans," are groups of cells in your pancreas. Islets contain several types of cells, including beta cells that make the hormone insulin. Insulin helps your body use glucose for energy and helps control your blood glucose levels, also called "blood sugar."

PANCREATIC ISLET TRANSPLANTATION

Pancreatic islet transplantation is an experimental treatment for type 1 diabetes. In this procedure, doctors take islets with healthy beta cells from the pancreas of a deceased organ donor and inject them into a vein that carries blood to the liver of a person with type 1 diabetes. These islets begin to make and release insulin in the recipient's body. More than one injection of transplanted islet cells is often needed to stop using insulin.

Researchers hope that islet transplantation will help people with type 1 diabetes:

- improve their blood glucose levels
- lower or remove the need for insulin injections
- better recognize symptoms of low blood glucose, also called "hypoglycemia"
- prevent severe hypoglycemia, which is when a person's blood glucose level becomes so low that she or he needs help from another person to treat the hypoglycemia

CANDIDATES FOR ISLET TRANSPLANTATION

Not all people with type 1 diabetes are good candidates for islet transplantation. Certain people with type 1 diabetes who have blood glucose levels that are difficult to manage, experience severe hypoglycemia, and have hypoglycemia unawareness—a dangerous condition in which a person cannot feel or recognize the symptoms of hypoglycemia—may be candidates.

Doctors consider people for islet transplantation if the possible benefits, such as being better able to reach blood glucose targets without problems like hypoglycemia, outweigh the risks, such as the possible side effects of immunosuppressants.

ISLET TRANSPLANTATION PROCEDURE

Special enzymes are used to remove islets from the pancreas of a deceased donor. The islets are purified and counted in a lab. On average, about 400,000 islets are transplanted in each procedure.

The recipient will most often receive a local anesthetic and a sedative—medicine to help them relax—for the procedure. In some cases, the recipient may receive general anesthesia.

The islet transplant infusion procedure involves inserting a thin, flexible tube called a "catheter" through a small cut in the recipient's upper abdomen. A radiologist uses x-rays and ultrasound to guide the catheter into the portal vein of the liver. The islets are slowly infused through the catheter and into the liver by gravity. Alternatively, a minimally invasive open procedure can directly visualize a vein near the liver to insert the catheter.

Over the next two weeks, new blood vessels form and connect the islets with the blood vessels of the recipient. The beta cells in the islets begin to make and release insulin into the bloodstream immediately after transplant.

BENEFITS OF ISLET TRANSPLANTATION

Recipients may see the following benefits:

- improved blood glucose levels
- less need or no need for insulin injections to manage diabetes
- fewer or no episodes of severe hypoglycemia
- improved awareness of hypoglycemia, which helps prevent episodes of severe hypoglycemia

Research also suggests that islet transplantation may prevent or slow the development of diabetes complications such as heart disease, kidney disease, and nerve or eye damage.

SUCCESS OF ISLET TRANSPLANTATION

A Phase 3 clinical trial conducted by the National Institutes of Health (NIH)-sponsored Clinical Islet Transplantation Consortium found that one year after islet transplantation, nearly 9 in 10 transplant recipients had an A1C level below 7 percent and did not have episodes of severe hypoglycemia. About half of the recipients did not need to take any insulin. Two years after islet transplantation, about 7 in 10 recipients had an A1C level of less than 7 percent and did not have episodes of severe hypoglycemia, and about 4 in 10 did not need insulin.

RISKS OF ISLET TRANSPLANTATION

Risks of islet transplantation include:

- bleeding, blood clots, and pain after the procedure
- the chance that the transplanted islets may not work well or may stop working
- side effects of antirejection medicines, also called "immunosuppressants"
- development of antibodies against the donor cells that may make it more difficult to find an appropriate organ donor if another transplant is needed in the future

OTHER USES OF ISLET TRANSPLANTATION

Doctors may perform a different type of islet transplantation, called "islet auto-transplantation," in people who have their whole pancreas removed to treat severe and chronic pancreatitis. In islet auto-transplantation, doctors remove a patient's pancreas, extract the islets, and transplant them into the patient's liver. The goal is to provide enough healthy islets to make insulin. Patients do not need to take immunosuppressants after islet auto-transplantation because they receive islets from their own bodies. Islet auto-transplantation is not considered experimental.[2]

[2] "Pancreatic Islet Transplantation," National Institute of Diabetes and Digestive and Kidney Diseases (NIDDK), October 2018. Available online. URL: www.niddk.nih.gov/health-information/diabetes/overview/insulin-medicines-treatments/pancreatic-islet-transplantation. Accessed April 17, 2024.

Section 25.7 | **Organ Transplant for Children**

Your child needs a transplant. What now? The path to organ transplantation is a journey. Your family's transplant journey may begin when your doctor tells you that your child needs an organ transplant, or when you find out that your child suffers from end-stage organ disease.

There are seven basic steps in the process before and during the transplant:

1. Find a transplant hospital.
2. Get to know your transplant team.
3. Transplant evaluation.
4. The waitlist.
5. Waiting for a match.
6. The call (organ offer).
7. Transplant surgery.

Each of these steps is unique to your child's condition. Your child may have a chronic illness in which a transplant is planned for months or years in advance, or your child may have an acute illness and need an urgent transplant within days or weeks. In these cases, the first steps may be compressed and require quick decisions with the support of the transplant team.

FIND A TRANSPLANT HOSPITAL

A transplant hospital is a hospital with health-care providers who specialize in all aspects of transplant medicine. All transplant hospitals in the United States are part of the OPTN. Not all hospitals perform transplants, and not all transplant hospitals do pediatric transplants.

Your child's doctor can refer you to a transplant hospital that:

- specializes in your child's medical condition
- is most conveniently located for your child's and family's needs
- will work with your insurance

GET TO KNOW YOUR TRANSPLANT TEAM

The transplant team will oversee your child's care. Team members will help you care for your child's health issues, identify and create your support system, and work on your financial plan. Each transplant hospital is different, and so are the team members. These are some of the roles that you may find:

- **Transplant coordinator.** Assists and guides you and your family through the transplant process, is your family's point-person at most hospitals, and helps you meet requirements to add your child to the transplant waitlist.
- **Transplant doctors and nurses.** Manage your child's care and arrange for tests, and provide you and your child with specific transplant information.
- **Transplant surgeon.** Performs the operation when an organ is available.
- **Transplant administrator.** Works behind the scenes to manage the team.
- **Social worker.** Helps you find support and services during your child's hospital stay and provides letters for work or school, if needed.
- **Psychologist.** Helps a child find ways to cope and reduce stress during the transplant process, and works with a child on taking medications (particularly during teenage years)
- **Transplant pharmacist.** Works with your doctors and discusses your child's transplant medications with them, and helps you figure out how to ensure your child takes all required medications.
- **Registered dietitian nutritionist.** Cares for the patient before, during, and after transplant, develops nutrition support regimens (tube feeds and IV nutrition), and vitamin and mineral supplements because good nutrition status is vital for a successful transplant.
- **Financial coordinator.** Helps you create a plan to cover costs before, during, and after your child's transplant, advises you on insurance issues, helps you find financial

aid, and explains copay charges (a social worker also may perform some of these duties at your center).
- **Child life services staff.** Help children and families cope with chronic illness and hospital stays. They provide age-appropriate support, including medical play therapy, to explain the transplant process and help children deal with their feelings. They may also help arrange schooling options for children in the hospital.
- **Organ procurement organization (OPO) staff.** Identify potential deceased donors and get authorization for donation, and work with your hospital and the donor hospital during the matching and organ procurement process.

TRANSPLANT EVALUATION

Your transplant team will order medical tests and lab work to evaluate your child for a transplant. These include blood tests, tissue typing, organ-specific tests, and a complete health history. Other tests gauge psychological readiness and social support. Results will help the team decide if your child meets the criteria to be a transplant candidate at their hospital.

The team also will decide how to best manage your child's medical condition and when your child will be listed for an organ transplant.

THE WAITLIST

The transplant team looks at a range of medical, surgical, psychological, developmental, and social factors when listing a patient for organ transplantation. If your child is accepted as a candidate, the transplant hospital will place your child on the national OPTN waitlist. OPOs and your transplant hospital will work together to find a match. There is still a possibility that not every transplant candidate will receive an organ because deceased organs are a scarce resource.

If your child needs a liver, kidney, or lung, a living donor transplant is possible at some hospitals. If you, a family member, or a friend wants to be a living donor for your child, you should contact the transplant hospital for information on how to start the evaluation and testing for this process.

WAITING FOR A MATCH

Waiting for a match can be emotionally difficult for your child and family. Some patients wait for a transplant for several months or years. Make sure that your child has a consistent daily schedule during this time. If your child is waiting for a transplant at home, talk with your medical team and follow their guidance about activity limits. If a child is waiting for a transplant for an extended time in the hospital, talk to the child life specialist. The specialist will provide a schedule and activities appropriate for the child's age, developmental level, and psychosocial needs.

The transplant team will monitor a child's condition as they wait for an organ offer. Some children could become more ill and may need to wait in the hospital. If a child is already in the hospital, they may need to move to the intensive care unit (ICU) to wait.

THE CALL (ORGAN OFFER)

Your transplant team will contact you when an organ is available that is the best match for your child.

When you arrive at the transplant hospital, get ready for more tests to prepare your child for surgery. At this point, you and your child may feel excited, anxious, afraid, or peaceful. You may also grieve for the family who lost someone but feel grateful that your child will receive the gift of life. Donor information is confidential, and you would not receive details about the donor, such as sex or age.

You may find out that final tests show that the organ is not suitable for transplant. You and your child may be disappointed to leave the hospital without a transplant. Your transplant team will use only organs that will give your child the best chance for a good outcome, but this kind of uncertainty can be hard to handle. Your reactions might include anxiety, grief, guilt, depression, anger, and confusion, to name a few. You should lean on your transplant team to help you deal with your emotions. Your transplant coordinator, social worker, child life specialist, psychologist, chaplain, and other team members can help you find strength to support your child and family.

TRANSPLANT SURGERY

Each transplant is unique, but the surgery lasts four to nine hours. It may take even longer for patients to receive more than one organ. All patients are placed on a breathing machine (ventilator) for the operation, but many patients will need to stay on the breathing machine after surgery, too. Your child will likely spend time in the ICU (intermediate care unit).

Each patient recovers differently. Ask your transplant team when your child can expect to eat, walk, and return to normal activities after transplant.[1]

Section 25.8 | **Preventing Fungal Diseases**

As an organ transplant patient, you have new opportunities for a healthy and full life. However, you may also face new health challenges, including avoiding infections. Antirejection medication helps you accept the new organ by lowering your body's immune system response, but it can also put you at greater risk for fungal infections.

Many fungal diseases that are mild for most people can be life-threatening for individuals with certain risk factors. Some fungal diseases are known to affect only those with weakened immune systems. The immune system fights germs, including fungi, from attacking the body and helps prevent fungal infections. People with some medical conditions or taking certain medications can have weakened immune systems, making them more likely to get fungal diseases, have more severe infections, and have a harder time recovering.

[1] "Pediatric Transplants," Health Resources and Services Administration (HRSA), December 18, 2020. Available online. URL: https://optn.transplant.hrsa.gov/patients/about-transplantation/pediatric-transplants. Accessed July 1, 2024.

RISK FACTORS OF FUNGAL INFECTIONS

Certain treatments and medications can also increase risk, such as:

- organ transplants
- stem cell transplants
- long-term hospital stays
- corticosteroids
- high doses of antibiotics

Certain medical conditions increase the risk of fungal infections, including:

- cancer
- HIV/AIDS
- chronic lung disease

Different fungal diseases may have more specific risk factors. Some diseases have risk factors unrelated to the immune system, such as race, age, and pregnancy. Health equity factors, including where a person lives, their occupation, and access to care, also affect fungal disease risks.

PEOPLE AT INCREASED RISK

People with Organ Transplants

People who receive organ transplants need to take anti-rejection medications. These medications weaken the immune system so it does not attack the new organ. Some transplants, such as small bowel, lung, liver, and heart transplants, may increase risk more than others.

People with Stem Cell Transplants

Stem cell transplants increase the risk of fungal infections because they destroy and rebuild the immune system. People can have stem cell transplants using their own cells or cells from a donor. People who receive donor stem cells are at higher risk for infections. Like people who have organ transplants, donor stem cell recipients need to take anti-rejection medications. Stem cell recipients are also at risk for graft-versus-host disease (GvHD), where transplanted stem cells attack the host's body.

People with Cancer

Chemotherapy and radiation are essential treatments for people with cancer. While they destroy cancer cells, they can also lower white blood cell counts. The immune system relies on white blood cells to fight infections. The type of fungal infection and level of risk can depend on the type of cancer and chemotherapy treatment.

People in Health-Care Settings

Patients in health-care settings typically have weakened immune systems, at least temporarily. Reasons for hospitalization, such as being sick, receiving intensive treatment (like chemotherapy), and recovering from surgery, all weaken the immune system. Patients can get infected by fungi entering wounds or surgical sites. Medical devices, such as ventilators and catheters, can create pathways for fungi to enter the body and cause infections. Some common health-care-associated infections include invasive candidiasis (specifically candidemia), aspergillosis, and mucormycosis. Aspergillosis and mucormycosis have been linked to mold outbreaks in hospitals, although this is rare. Mold outbreaks can occur near construction sites, through contaminated ventilation systems, or in laundry. *Candida auris* (*C. auris*) is a fungus that can cause severe, often antifungal-resistant illness in hospitalized patients. Unlike other health-care-associated fungal infections, they spread easily and often cause outbreaks in health-care settings.

PREVENTION OF FUNGAL INFECTIONS

Environmental

It may not be possible to prevent exposure to some fungi that live in the environment. Fungi can release spores into the air we breathe. These steps may help lower risks:

- Find out if certain fungal diseases are common in your area (e.g., blastomycosis, histoplasmosis, or Valley fever).
- Avoid situations that increase exposure to dust, such as construction sites and dust storms.
- Wear long pants and long-sleeved shirts for outdoor activities.

Health-Care-Associated

People in health-care settings can learn about how to be a safe patient. Frequent handwashing is crucial for patients, visitors, and health-care providers.

CONSULTING A HEALTH-CARE PROVIDER

Health-care providers may prescribe antifungal medications to people at very high risk to help prevent fungal infections. Many fungal diseases are misdiagnosed. If you think you have a fungal infection or are being treated for an infection that is not improving, ask your health-care provider about testing and antifungal treatment.

By taking these precautions and being aware of the risks, you can help manage your health effectively after an organ transplant and reduce the likelihood of serious fungal infections.[1]

[1] "Risk Factors for Fungal Diseases," Centers for Disease Control and Prevention (CDC), May 8, 2024. Available online. URL: www.cdc.gov/fungal/risk-factors. Accessed July 16, 2024.

Chapter 26 | **Amputation Surgeries**

Chapter Contents

INFORMED CONSENT PROCESS

The informed consent process is essential to any surgical intervention and is legally required. The discussion before surgery is usually the first contact between the patient and the surgeon conducting the operation. This discussion provides an opportunity to form a trusting relationship and open communication to address patient's fears, wishes, and concerns. The surgeon must inform the patient about the risks and benefits of each viable treatment option. Patients should be encouraged to ask questions, express their personal desires, understand the options, and agree to a treatment plan before undertaking upper extremity amputation. Special consideration must be given in cases where the patient cannot consent to surgery.

The decision regarding amputation should be based on accepted surgical and medical standards of care. Surgeons should be familiar with the multiple approaches available for various amputation levels, muscle-balancing strategies, and wound closure techniques. Emerging and advanced surgical techniques may be performed in a specialized setting under the care of experienced surgeons. Combined with sophisticated medical and rehabilitation care, amputation surgeries can also serve as refined reconstructive procedures to prepare the residual limb not only for motor function but also for sensory feedback and cosmesis.

URGENT AMPUTATION SITUATIONS

Severe trauma, critical extremity ischemia, and/or overwhelming infection generally require urgent amputation surgery. An urgent amputation may also be necessary when vessel occlusion and subsequent extremity tissue necrosis result from using vasoconstrictor agents to treat infections (sepsis). In trauma cases where the immediate threat to life is not serious, a period of conservative management may be observed to monitor the evolution of the patient's condition. This period may allow for the restoration of collateral circulation in the extremity, potentially avoiding amputation or minimizing the segment to be removed. Emergency repair of torn blood vessels by the vascular surgeon can make extremities viable and help avoid amputation.

LIMB SALVAGE VERSUS AMPUTATION

Health-care providers should recognize that extensive reconstructive surgery to preserve an extremity may result in a painful, nonfunctional, and less efficient limb than an amputated limb with a prosthesis. Conversely, an upper limb with minimal function can sometimes be more useful than an amputation with a prosthesis. Therefore, careful consideration should be given to the decision about limb salvage versus amputation.

AMPUTATION FOR CANCER

When considering amputation as a treatment for cancer, the care team should involve the orthopedic oncology or general surgery oncology teams (if available) to add more subject expertise to the decision-making process. Elective or delayed amputations may be considered when the affected extremity is nonfunctional due to the loss of compensated vascular, neurologic, or musculoskeletal function, resulting in a significant decline in patient health, quality of life (QOL), and well-being. It is crucial that patients undergo a comprehensive mental health assessment to ensure sound decision-making capacity and a well-informed decision regarding elective or delayed amputation.

SURGICAL TECHNIQUE AND COLLABORATION

With any amputation surgery, consideration should be given to the surgical technique that will result in the highest level of functional ability, including available prosthesis treatment options. This can be accomplished through early consultations and collaboration with other care team members with subject expertise (prosthetist, physiatrist, etc.). This collaboration provides the best opportunity for the patient to achieve maximal postsurgical function and outcomes.

PRIMARY GOAL OF AMPUTATION

The primary goal of amputation is to remove the diseased, damaged, or dysfunctional portion of the limb while ensuring the residual limb is optimized for motion, motion control, and proprioceptive feedback to achieve the most successful outcomes. In general, maximum preservation of length is desirable in upper limb amputation. Preserving joints and limb length enhances the patient's ability to position the residual limb and/or prosthetic device in space, allowing optimal functional results and improved outcomes.

However, there may be instances when preserving maximal limb length would hinder functional outcomes with a prosthesis, thereby limiting functional independence. These situations should be thoroughly discussed with the surgeon and care team. In traumatic amputation cases, the scope of injury often determines the amputation level. In cases of vascular disease, the level of amputation is often dictated by blood flow and tissue viability. It is important for the surgeon to understand the requirements and capabilities of available prostheses for each amputation level, allotransplantation, and other evolving treatments to direct opportunities for limb length preservation when available.

SURGICAL LEVELS AND CONSIDERATIONS

Consider surgeons who:

- Do not perform guillotine-style amputation.
- Complete the amputation within the zone of injury to maximize length.
- Preserve at least 5 cm of humerus length to maintain a transhumeral amputation level.
- Preserve at least 5 cm of ulnar length to maintain a transradial amputation.
- Special consideration for disarticulation at the elbow or wrist level, partial hand amputation, and other complex or unusual cases.
- Perform myogenesis for all primary-function muscles. Myoplasty and myofascial closure may be used to secure secondary muscles and contour muscles for final amputation closure.

- Use skin grafts and dermal substitutes to allow amputation closure if a primary fasciocutaneous closure is unavailable.[1]

Section 26.2 | **Lower Limb Amputation**

DYSVASCULAR AMPUTATION

In civilian and elderly U.S. Department of Veterans Affairs (VA) populations, the most common cause of lower limb amputation (LLA) is dysvascular complications from diabetes, arteriosclerosis, smoking, or a combination of these factors. Amputation may occur when medical or revascularization options do not exist or have failed, when significant tissue loss has occurred, or when infectious complications can only be managed surgically. In diabetic patients, protective and prophylactic foot care and early detection of deformities or skin breakdown can prevent ulcers and reduce the risk of amputation. Smoking cessation and control of cardiovascular risk factors, including glycemic control in diabetics, are additional approaches to preventing LLA. Due to the systemic nature of arteriosclerosis and diabetes, patients with these conditions are at high risk for further complications to their amputated residual limb and/or amputation of the contralateral limb. They are also at higher risk for other health problems such as cardiovascular disease (CVD), cerebrovascular accident, renal disease, and peripheral neuropathy. Preservation of the residual and contralateral limb, as well as the patient's general health, wellness, and functional independence, remain integral parts of ongoing care.

TRAUMATIC AMPUTATION

Trauma is another major cause of LLA, though not as common as dysvascular amputations. Traumatic amputation may result from

[1] "VA/DoD Clinical Practice Guideline for the Management of Upper Extremity Amputation Rehabilitation," U.S. Department of Veterans Affairs (VA), 2014. Available online. URL: www.healthquality.va.gov/guidelines/Rehab/UEAR/VADoDCPGManagementofUEAR121614Corrected508.pdf. Accessed July 9, 2024.

motor vehicle and industrial accidents, electrical, chemical, and thermal burns, and injuries associated with power tools or heavy machinery use. Military and veteran populations are particularly concerned with amputations related to combat injuries, such as those from explosions or crush injuries. These injuries are often complicated by other conditions, including traumatic brain injury, posttraumatic stress, and other soft tissue injuries.

OTHER CAUSES OF AMPUTATION

Other less prevalent causes of amputation include malignant musculoskeletal tumors, infection, iatrogenic complications of vascular access procedures for other medical problems, and congenital limb development deficiency. The goal in treating musculoskeletal tumors with a low risk of recurrence is to remove the tumor and salvage the limb. For tumors with a high risk of local recurrence or metastasis, amputation is often indicated. Treatment of infection may require amputation when initial treatment leads to vessel occlusion and extremity necrosis. Chronic or recurring infection after total knee arthroplasty may also lead to transfemoral amputation. Congenital limb deficiencies account for a small percentage of lower limb loss, and definitive amputation is performed at a time that considers skeletal growth and supports physical, behavioral, and psychological development.

LIMB SALVAGE AND DELAYED AMPUTATION

For severe limb injury, patients and surgeons often face the decision between amputation and limb reconstruction and salvage. While limb salvage may initially be the therapeutic option of choice, complications such as infection, chronic pain, or persistent dysfunction may result in delayed amputation. Limb salvage decisions may lead to increased complications, pain, and procedures compared to primary amputation. To mitigate these risks, scoring systems have been developed to assist with the decision to amputate or salvage the limb, but they may not accurately predict functional recovery. Unsuccessful limb salvage attempts may result in increased morbidity and mortality. Studies have shown greater hospitalization days and more operative procedures for individuals who underwent delayed versus primary amputation surgery. Additionally, service members with combat-related amputations demonstrated better functional outcomes compared to those with limb salvage.[1]

THE APPROPRIATE LEVEL OF SURGERY

Once the patient is optimized for surgery, the surgeon must determine the level of amputation. This decision will affect the patient's rehabilitation, functional outcome, and long-term quality of life. Factors considered include the patient and family perspective, input from the rehabilitation team, and principles of amputation surgery.

Optimal Residual Limb Length

TRANSTIBIAL AMPUTATION

- **Optimum.** Length that allows space for the prosthetic foot and sufficient muscle padding—typically mid-tibia.
- **Minimum.** Junction of the middle third and proximal third of the tibia, just below the tibial plateau, to allow sufficient tibia for weight-bearing.

TRANSFEMORAL AMPUTATION

- **Optimum.** Length that allows space for an uncompromising knee system—typically just above the condylar flair.
- **Minimum.** Junction of the middle third and proximal third (below the level of the lesser trochanter) to allow sufficient femur length/lever arm to operate the prosthesis.

If there is uncertainty about the optimal length of the residual limb, preoperative consultation with an experienced physiatrist or prosthetist should be considered.

---

[1] "VA/DoD Clinical Practice Guideline for Rehabilitation of Individuals with Lower Limb Amputation," U.S. Department of Veterans Affairs (VA), 2017. Available online. URL: www.healthquality.va.gov/guidelines/Rehab/amp/VADoDLLACPG092817.pdf. Accessed July 9, 2024.

POTENTIAL FOR WOUND HEALING

The potential for wound healing should be determined through laboratory studies, imaging studies, and additional tests.

Laboratory Studies

- **C-reactive protein**. To check for infection.
- **Hemoglobin**. To check for treatable anemia and ensure appropriate oxygenation for wound healing.
- **Absolute lymphocyte count**. To check for immune deficiency and/or infection.
- **Serum albumin/prealbumin level**. To check for malnutrition and diminished ability to heal.

Imaging Studies

- **Radiography**. Anteroposterior and lateral views of the involved extremity.
- **CT scan and MRI**. As necessary.
- **Doppler ultrasonography**. To measure arterial pressure.

Additional Tests

- **Ischemic index (II)**. Ratio of Doppler pressure at the level being tested to brachial systolic pressure—a II of 0.5 or greater supports healing.
- **$TcPO_2$ levels**. Preoperative levels greater than 20 mmHg are associated with successful healing after amputation.

BALANCING FACTORS FOR AMPUTATION LEVEL

Determining the optimum amputation level involves balancing the patient's goals and expectations, risks associated with additional surgery, functional and cardiovascular consequences of more proximal amputations, surgeons' clinical experience, and the physiological potential for the residual limb to heal. Other factors include cosmesis, mobility goals, and specialized vocational or recreational priorities. The ultimate functional desires and expectations of the patient need to be included in the decision-making process.

Due to the patient's underlying comorbid cardiovascular disease, increased energy expenditure may result in a lower level of function and possibly no ambulation. The level of amputation is more predictive of mobility than other factors such as age, sex, diabetes, emergency admission, indication for amputation, and previous vascular surgery. The decision must also consider the reason for the amputation (e.g., disease process, trauma), the vascular supply to the skin flaps, and the required limb fitting procedures and techniques available.

Amputation should preserve as much of the limb as possible, as the longer the lever arm, the more control a patient will have over a prosthesis. Preserving the knee can decrease the energy consumption required for ambulating. In transtibial amputations, increased energy expenditure in walking is 25–40 percent above normal, while in transfemoral amputations, it is 68–100 percent above normal. Therefore, patients with transtibial amputations usually have better mobility than those with transfemoral amputations. The site of injury largely determines the decision regarding the level of the section. Ensuring the residual limb is covered with skin that has normal sensation and is free of scar tissue as much as possible and that the end of the residual limb is adequately covered with muscles is crucial for successful outcomes.[2]

Section 26.3 | **Postamputation Pain and Other Complications**

RESIDUAL LIMB CARE

Following amputation, the residual limb undergoes numerous changes over time, potentially resulting in secondary complications and limiting the ability to wear a prosthesis for functional activities. These changes and complications include:

- soft tissue and muscle atrophy
- skin irritation and breakdown
- joint contracture

[2] "VA/DoD Clinical Practice Guideline for Rehabilitation of Lower Limb Amputation," U.S. Department of Veterans Affairs (VA), 2007. Available online. URL: www.healthquality.va.gov/guidelines/rehab/amp/amp_v652.pdf. Accessed July 9, 2024.

- infection (soft tissue and bone)
- proximal osteoarthritis/musculoskeletal complications
- heterotopic ossification
- osteopenia and osteoporosis

PAIN MANAGEMENT

Pain following amputation can generally be classified as residual limb pain or phantom limb pain.

Residual Limb Pain

Typically, improves following amputation surgery but can be persistent and associated with prosthetic use.

Phantom Limb Pain

Pain is perceived in the part of the body that is missing. This pain can be chronic and severe enough to interfere with prosthetic use and functional abilities.

OTHER TRAUMATIC INJURY CONSIDERATIONS

Amputations related to combat and other trauma are commonly associated with moderate to severe injury severity scores and multiple comorbid injuries requiring long-term management and care. These associated injuries can affect medical and rehabilitation outcomes such as functional independence, satisfaction, and quality of life (QOL). Frequently associated injuries include:

- traumatic brain injury (TBI)
- fractures and other musculoskeletal injuries
- soft tissue injuries and burns
- peripheral nerve injuries
- abdominal injuries
- hearing loss and tinnitus
- vision impairment or loss
- genitourinary injuries (common with dismounted blast explosions)
- mental health conditions such as posttraumatic stress disorder (PTSD), depression, and adjustment disorder

SECONDARY COMPLICATIONS

Amputation of one or more limbs has a longitudinal effect on many areas outside the residual limb. The two areas most commonly affected are the musculoskeletal and cardiovascular systems. Many considerations in these areas gradually progress or worsen, while others may be more intermittent. Comprehensive prevention strategies, including proper nutrition, exercise, tobacco cessation, and wellness counseling, are crucial for individuals with amputations. Wellness promotion and preventive measures should be part of one's lifestyle. Medical monitoring and education should be routine in amputation clinics and rehabilitation services.

Musculoskeletal Considerations

Longitudinal considerations for musculoskeletal conditions include:

- osteoarthritis in the nonamputated extremity
- overuse syndromes
- delayed amputation after initial limb salvage
- general musculoskeletal pain and low back pain

Weight Gain/Obesity

Decreased activity levels and metabolic changes can result in weight gain and obesity. This weight gain can lead to a vicious cycle where weight gain makes prosthetic fitting and use more difficult, thus resulting in even greater declines in activity.

Cardiovascular Disease

The aging amputee population has significantly worse cardiovascular and metabolic issues directly related to their traumatic amputation, not accounted for by obesity, sedentary lifestyle, or tobacco use. Persons with traumatic amputations have been identified as having increased hypertension, ischemic heart disease, and diabetes mellitus. Lower extremity amputees should be monitored for aortic aneurysms, which occur at a reported rate of 6 percent versus 1 percent in the nonamputee population.[1]

---

[1] "Amputation System of Care Traumatic Amputation," U.S. Department of Veterans Affairs (VA), May 7, 2014. Available online. URL: www.prosthetics.va.gov/factsheet/ASoC_Traumatic_Amputation_Fact_Sheet_Short_Version_Sec_508_9_20_12.pdf. Accessed July 9, 2024

Chapter 27 | **Understanding Plastic and Reconstructive Surgery**

CATEGORIES OF PLASTIC SURGERY

According to the American Society of Plastic Surgeons (ASPS), the specialty of plastic surgery encompasses two main categories: cosmetic surgery and reconstructive surgery.

- **Cosmetic surgery**. Performed to reshape and adjust normal body structures to enhance visual appearance.
- **Reconstructive surgery**. Performed to restore and improve function and correct deformities or abnormal structures caused by congenital defects, developmental abnormalities, trauma, infection, tumors, or disease.

PROCEDURES AND INDICATIONS

Dermabrasion

DESCRIPTION

Dermabrasion is a skin resurfacing technique used to remove damaged skin and promote normal wound healing and skin rejuvenation. Standard dermabrasion uses a wire brush or a stainless steel wheel with diamond chips, while laser dermabrasion employs lasers such as the argon laser, ultrapulse CO_2 laser, or flashlamp-pumped pulsed dye laser.

MEDICAL NECESSITY

Dermabrasion is considered medically reasonable and necessary for treating rhinophyma, characterized by skin thickening and nasal enlargement due to excess tissue and sebaceous gland overgrowth. Rhinophyma can cause functional problems such as nasal airway obstruction and sleep apnea.

Abdominal Lipectomy/Panniculectomy

DESCRIPTION

These procedures involve the surgical removal of excessive fat and skin from the abdomen without muscle plication or flap elevation.

MEDICAL NECESSITY

Abdominal lipectomy/panniculectomy is considered medically reasonable and necessary when the pannus or panniculus hangs below the symphysis pubis, causing chronic intertrigo, difficulty walking, or functional impairment in daily activities. Additional criteria include maintaining stable weight for at least six months post-weight loss surgery.

Reconstructive Breast Surgery: Removal of Breast Implants

DESCRIPTION

This procedure aims to restore the normal appearance of a breast after mastectomy or to address complications related to breast implants.

MEDICAL NECESSITY

Removal of breast implants is considered medically reasonable and necessary for conditions such as broken or failed implants, infection, implant extrusion, siliconoma or granuloma, interference with breast cancer diagnosis, and painful capsular contracture with disfigurement.

Reduction Mammaplasty

DESCRIPTION

Reduction mammaplasty involves reducing breast size to alleviate symptoms caused by macromastia (breast hypertrophy).

MEDICAL NECESSITY

Reduction mammaplasty is considered medically reasonable and necessary when breast hypertrophy causes symptoms that have not responded to nonsurgical interventions. Symptoms include back pain, shoulder grooving, significant arthritic changes, and dermatologic issues. The procedure is also necessary to achieve symmetry with a reconstructed breast post-cancer surgery.

Mastectomy for Gynecomastia

DESCRIPTION

Gynecomastia surgery involves the removal of enlarged male breast tissue.

MEDICAL NECESSITY

Mastectomy for gynecomastia is considered reconstructive and medically necessary for males with Grade III or IV gynecomastia, persistent symptoms after medical treatment, pain affecting daily activities, and significant clinical manifestations affecting the supporting structures of the shoulders, neck, and trunk.

Rhinoplasty/Reconstructive Nasal Surgery

DESCRIPTION

Nasal surgery involves procedures on the external or internal structures of the nose, septum, or turbinate to improve function, correct deformities, or enhance appearance.

MEDICAL NECESSITY

Rhinoplasty and septoplasty are considered medically reasonable and necessary for correcting nasal deformities due to congenital craniofacial deformities, chronic nasal obstruction, trauma, disease, or secondary issues not resolved by septoplasty/turbinectomy alone. Septoplasty is indicated for nasal airway obstruction unresponsive to conservative treatment, recurrent sinusitis, recurrent epistaxis, and as part of cleft lip or palate repair.

COVERED INDICATIONS

Dermabrasion

- treatment of rhinophyma causing functional problems such as nasal airway obstruction and sleep apnea

Abdominal Lipectomy/Panniculectomy

- chronic intertrigo refractory to medical therapy for over three months
- difficulty walking or functional impairment in daily activities
- stable weight for at least six months post-weight loss surgery

Reconstructive Breast Surgery: Removal of Breast Implants

- broken or failed implants
- infection or inflammatory reaction due to breast prosthesis
- implant extrusion
- siliconoma or granuloma
- interference with breast cancer diagnosis
- painful capsular contracture with disfigurement

Reduction Mammaplasty

- symptoms unresponsive to non-surgical interventions
- dermatologic issues refractory to medical treatment
- back pain unrelieved by conservative measures
- shoulder grooving with skin irritation
- arthritic changes with persistent symptoms
- symmetry with reconstructed breast post-cancer surgery

Mastectomy for Gynecomastia

- persistent symptoms after medical treatment for pathological gynecomastia
- pain or tenderness affecting daily activities
- clinical symptoms refractory to analgesics or anti-inflammatory agents

- significant clinical manifestations affecting supporting structures

Rhinoplasty/Reconstructive Nasal Surgery

- correction of nasal deformities secondary to congenital craniofacial deformities or trauma
- chronic nasal obstruction due to vestibular stenosis
- nasal airway obstruction unresponsive to conservative treatment
- recurrent sinusitis secondary to septal deformity
- recurrent epistaxis related to septal deformity
- as part of cleft lip or palate repair

LIMITATIONS

The following procedures are considered cosmetic and not covered by Medicare:

- **Dermabrasion**. For post acne scarring, rosacea (other than rhinophyma), and other indications not covered above.
- **Abdominal lipectomy/panniculectomy**. For improving appearance, repairing abdominal wall laxity, or diastasis recti without chronic infection or inflammation.
- **Reconstructive breast surgery**. For reshaping breasts for appearance or self-image improvement, and reimplantation of cosmetic-only implants.
- **Reduction mammaplasty**. For reshaping breasts for appearance or self-image improvement, and mammopexy unrelated to breast reconstruction postmastectomy.
- **Mastectomy for gynecomastia**. As the first line of treatment or solely to improve appearance or alter chest wall contours.
- **Gigantomastia of pregnancy**. For reshaping breasts for appearance or self-image improvement.
- **Rhinoplasty/reconstructive nasal surgery**. Solely to alter appearance or improve self-image without

functional abnormalities, or as the primary treatment for obstructive sleep disorder without meeting listed indications.[1]

[1] "Plastic Surgery," Centers for Medicare & Medicaid Services (CMS), April 2, 2020. Available online. URL: www.cms.gov/medicare-coverage-database/view/lcd.aspx?LCDId=37020&ContrId=345. Accessed July 8, 2024.

Chapter 28 | Surgery for Gender Dysphoria

UNDERSTANDING GENDER DYSPHORIA

Gender dysphoria involves a discrepancy between a person's gender identity and their sex assigned at birth. This can cause significant distress and lead to higher rates of depression and anxiety. Treatment is tailored to each individual and may include a combination of psychotherapy, hormone therapy, and surgical interventions. The primary goal of treatment is to alleviate distress and help individuals live comfortably in their desired gender role.

BENEFITS OF GENDER-AFFIRMING SURGERIES

Gender-affirming surgeries (GAS) have shown significant benefits in numerous studies over the past several decades. These surgeries are generally safe, effective, and necessary for many individuals experiencing gender dysphoria. Feelings of regret are extremely rare and typically temporary. Access to gender-affirming care improves psychological outcomes and overall health.

INDIVIDUALIZED TREATMENT PLANS

The purpose of gender-affirming treatments, whether surgical or hormonal, is to address gender dysphoria and improve overall well-being. Each patient's treatment plan should be individualized, considering the totality of their needs and appearance. Transgender individuals have unique clinical needs that differ from nontransgender individuals, and assessments should be based on their specific symptoms and goals.

CATEGORIES OF GENDER-AFFIRMING SURGERY

Gender-affirming surgeries can be categorized as follows:

- breast/chest surgeries
- genital surgeries
- other surgeries

For transgender men, these procedures may include:

- **Breast/chest surgery**. Subcutaneous mastectomy, nipple grafts, chest reconstruction.
- **Genital surgery**. Hysterectomy/salpingo-oophorectomy, metoidioplasty, phalloplasty (using a pedicled or free vascularized flap), reconstruction of the fixed part of the urethra, vaginectomy, vulvectomy, scrotoplasty, and implantation of erection and/or testicular prostheses.
- **Other surgeries**. Voice surgery (rare), liposuction, and lipofilling.

For transgender women, these procedures may include:

- **Breast/chest surgery**. Mammaplasty.
- **Genital surgery**. Orchiectomy, penectomy, vaginoplasty, clitoroplasty, vulvoplasty, labiaplasty, urethroplasty, and rarely prostatectomy.
- **Other surgeries**. Reconstructive facial feminization surgery, liposuction, lipofilling, voice surgery, thyroid cartilage reduction, electrolysis or laser hair removal, and hair reconstruction.

SURGERIES FOR TRANSGENDER MEN

Breast/Chest Surgery

Mastectomy for transgender men is often necessary to alleviate gender dysphoria. Both double-incision mastectomy with nipple grafts and keyhole mastectomy are effective procedures. Reconstruction of the chest to approximate a typical male appearance is a necessary component.

Genital Surgeries

Hysterectomy (with or without salpingectomy and oophorectomy), metoidioplasty, and phalloplasty are effective in treating gender dysphoria. These procedures have acceptable complication rates and can significantly improve quality of life (QOL). Scrotoplasty and testicular implants may also be necessary.

SURGERIES FOR TRANSGENDER WOMEN

Breast/Chest Surgery

In transgender women undergoing hormone therapy, breast development may be insufficient. In such cases, breast reconstruction is necessary and should be considered a reconstructive procedure rather than cosmetic. It has been shown to improve psychosocial well-being and reduce gender dysphoria.

Genital Surgeries

Orchiectomy and vaginoplasty are common procedures for transgender women. These surgeries are effective in treating gender dysphoria and have high satisfaction rates. Complications are generally manageable and outweighed by the benefits.

Other Surgeries

Facial and body hair removal, reconstructive facial feminization surgery, reduction thyroid chondroplasty, vocal surgery, and hair reconstruction may be necessary for many transgender women. These procedures are not cosmetic but reconstructive, helping individuals navigate the world as their true gender.

Facial feminization surgery is highly effective and associated with high satisfaction rates. It helps transgender women be perceived as female, reducing gender-based violence and discrimination. Hair removal through electrolysis or laser treatments is also necessary for many transgender women.[1]

---

[1] "Summary of Clinical Evidence for Gender Reassignment Surgeries," Centers for Medicare & Medicaid Services (CMS), January 2, 2016. Available online. URL: www.cms.gov/Medicare/Coverage/DeterminationProcess/Downloads/Kalra_comment_01022016_b.pdf. Accessed July 9, 2024.

Part 4 | Managing Postoperative Pain and Complications

Chapter 29 | **Pain Management after Surgery**

WHAT IS PAIN?

Pain is an uncomfortable feeling that signals something may be wrong in your body. When there is an injury (e.g., surgery, broken bones) or a painful disease or condition (e.g., sickle cell disease, arthritis, cancer), tiny nerve cells send messages to your brain. Pain medicine blocks or lessens these messages.

WHY IS PAIN CONTROL IMPORTANT?

Pain can affect your activity, appetite, sleep, energy, mood, and relationships. It can also affect your rate of recovery from surgery. Pain relief allows you to start walking and doing breathing exercises, so you can regain your strength faster and leave the hospital sooner. It helps you avoid problems such as pneumonia and blood clots, provides greater comfort while you heal, and may help you heal faster.

CAN PAIN BE RELIEVED?

Pain, in almost all cases, can be controlled. Although pain is common after surgery and with many types of illness, most patients with postoperative pain can be kept comfortable with simple treatment.

WILL YOU BECOME ADDICTED TO THE PAIN MEDICINE?

It is very unlikely that you will become addicted to pain medication when used as prescribed by your physician. Studies have shown that becoming addicted to pain medication is rare unless you already have a problem with substance abuse.

MEDICINES FOR PAIN RELIEF

Nonsteroidal Anti-inflammatory Drugs (NSAIDs)

- Acetaminophen (e.g., Tylenol) relieves mild-to-moderate pain and soreness.
- Aspirin and ibuprofen (e.g., Motrin) reduce swelling and soreness and relieve mild-to-moderate pain.
- Benefits:
  - These medicines can lessen or eliminate the need for stronger medicines (e.g., morphine or another opioid).
- Risks:
  - Most NSAIDs interfere with blood clotting. They may cause nausea, stomach bleeding, or kidney problems. For severe pain, an opioid usually must be added.

Opioids

- Morphine, oxycodone, codeine, and other opioids are most often used for acute pain, such as short-term pain after surgery.
- Benefits:
  - Effective for severe pain; do not cause bleeding in the stomach or elsewhere. It is rare for a patient to become addicted as a result of taking opioids for postoperative pain.
- Risks:
  - It may cause drowsiness, nausea, constipation, itching, or interfere with breathing or urination.

Local Anesthetics

- Bupivacaine is given either near the incision, near nerves, or through a small tube in your back to block the nerves that transmit pain signals.

- Benefits:
  - Effective for severe pain. Injections or infusions at the incision site block pain from that site. There is little or no risk of drowsiness, constipation, or breathing problems. Local anesthetics reduce the need for opioid use.
- Risks:
  - Repeated injections or continuous infusions are needed to maintain pain relief. Average epidural doses may cause some patients to have weakness in their legs or dizziness.

HOW ARE PAIN MEDICINES GIVEN?

Oral Medication

- Pills (tablets or capsules) and liquid that are taken by mouth.
- Benefits:
  - They cause less discomfort than injections into muscle or fat, and they can work just as well. They are inexpensive, simple to give, and easy to use at home.
- Risks:
  - It cannot be used if nothing can be taken by mouth or if you are nauseated or vomiting. There may be a delay in pain relief since you must ask for the medicine and wait for it to be brought to you. These medicines take time (30–60 minutes) to take full effect.

Intramuscular or Subcutaneous

- An injection of medicine that is given into a muscle or fat.
- Benefits:
  - It is effective even if you are nauseated or vomiting. It is simple to give, does not require intravenous (IV) access, and successfully controls moderate to severe pain in all regions of the body.
- Risks:
  - The injection site is usually painful for a short time. There is a possibility of infection, sterile abscess, or peripheral

nerve injury. It is more expensive than tablets or liquids. Pain relief may be delayed while you ask the nurse for medicine and wait for the shot to be drawn up and given. Due to the variable absorption and the time and staff necessary to administer, other routes are preferred.

Patient-Controlled Analgesia or Intravenous

- An injection of medication that is given into a vein. IV patient-controlled analgesia (PCA) allows you to control when you get IV pain medication. When you begin to feel pain, you press a button to inject the pain medicine through the IV into your vein.
- Benefits:
    - Medication is fully absorbed, and acts quickly. Well suited for the relief of brief episodes of pain. When an IV PCA pump is used, you can control your doses of pain medicine.
- Risks:
    - A small tube must be inserted in a vein. You must want to use the pump and learn how and when to give yourself doses of medicine if you use IV PCA.

Regional Analgesia

- Local anesthetic injections along a nerve provide pain relief to a specific area of the body and decrease systemic side effects.
- Benefits:
    - Limiting the analgesia to a body region may allow for reducing or eliminating other types of pain medication. Reducing the need for other types of pain medication may reduce the incidence of adverse effects.
- Risks:
    - It requires knowledgeable providers and specialized equipment. If a single administration is used, the duration of action is limited, so patients may also require some other methods of pain relief.

Epidural or Spinal

- Medication is given by injection or through a small tube placed in your back (epidural space or into the spinal fluid). The tube may be connected to a pump, which delivers pain medicine. Some pumps allow you to press a button to inject the pain medicine, while others provide a continuous flow of medication.
- Benefits:
  - Works well when you have chest surgery or an operation on the lower parts of your body. Provides excellent pain relief with minimal side effects from the medications because they are given in lower doses.
- Risks:
  - Staff must be specially trained to place a small tube in the back and to watch for problems that can appear hours after pain medicine is given. A spinal anesthetic may only provide relief for the duration of the operation, and you may require medications by other routes after the operation. You may not be allowed to walk or may be required to walk with assistance only while an epidural catheter is in place. You may also experience difficulty urinating, which may require a urinary catheter to be placed.

Rectal

- Medication in a suppository is placed into the rectum.
- Benefits:
  - Inexpensive, simple to give, and easy to use at home.
- Risks:
  - Some people do not like this route. There may be a delay in pain relief since you must ask for the medicine and wait for it to be brought to you. These medicines take time (30–60 minutes) to take full effect.

NONDRUG MEASURES FOR PAIN RELIEF

Education

- Learning about the operation and the pain expected afterward may reduce anxiety and pain.
- Benefits:
  - Reduces anxiety; no equipment needed.
- Risks:
  - No risks, but patient attention and cooperation with staff are required

Relaxation

- Simple techniques such as abdominal breathing and jaw relaxation can help increase comfort after surgery.
- Benefits:
  - Easy to learn, reduces anxiety, can be used at any time, no equipment needed.
- Risks:
  - No risks, but instruction from a health-care provider is needed

Slow Rhythmic Breathing for Relaxation

- Breathe in slowly and deeply.
- As you breathe out slowly, feel yourself beginning to relax; feel the tension leaving your body.
- Now, breathe in and out slowly and regularly, at whatever rate is comfortable for you. You may wish to try abdominal breathing. If you do not know how to do abdominal breathing, ask your nurse for help.
- To help you focus on breathing slowly and rhythmically, Breathe in as you silently say, "In, two, three." Breathe out as you silently say, "Out, two, three."
- Each time you breathe out, silently say a word such as "peace" or "relax."
- You may imagine that you are doing this in a place that is very calming and relaxing, such as lying in the sun at the beach.

- Do steps 1 through 4 only once, or repeat steps 3 and 4 for up to 20 minutes.
- End with a slow, deep breath. As you breathe out, say to yourself, "I feel alert and relaxed."
- If you intend to do this for over a few seconds, try to get in a comfortable position in a quiet place. You may close your eyes or focus on an object. This breathing exercise may be used for only a few seconds or up to 20 minutes.

Physical Agents

- Cold packs, support of the surgical site while moving, and mild exercises such as walking, massage, rest, heat, and transcutaneous electrical nerve stimulation (TENS) are some nondrug pain relief methods that might be used following surgery.
- Benefits:
  - In general, physical agents are safe and have no side effects. They act quickly and can be controlled by the patient. Walking is very beneficial in relieving gas pains.
- Risks:
  - Few risks are related to the use of physical techniques. Your physician should approve the use of heat or cold after surgery. If TENS is used, there is some cost and staff time involved in purchasing the machine and instructing patients in its use.

Distraction

- Distraction prevents or lessens the perception of pain by focusing attention on sensations unrelated to pain. The goals of distraction are to increase pain tolerance and perceived control and decrease pain intensity. This technique can involve all the senses.
- Benefits:
  - It is safe, has no side effects, can be individualized to each person's interests, and can include music, videos, reading, humor, and television.

- Risks:
    - No risks.

Hypnosis

- A state of focused attention allows distraction from external stimuli. The induction of this state has been shown to improve pain management.
- Benefits:
    - Safe, decreases anxiety.
- Risks:
    - Requires a professional trained in hypnosis to assist with this procedure. It does not work with all patients.[1]

[1] "VHA/DoD Clinical Practice Guideline for the Management of Postoperative Pain," U.S. Department of Veterans Affairs (VA), May 2002. Available online. URL: www.healthquality.va.gov/guidelines/Pain/pop/pop_fulltext.pdf. Accessed April 8, 2024.

Chapter 30 | **Postoperative Hemorrhage Prevention and Management**

ESSENTIAL FIRST STEPS

Preoperative, perioperative, and procedure personnel—including nurses, physicians, other providers, surgical technicians, and representatives from the quality improvement department—develop evidence-based protocols for patient care to prevent postoperative hemorrhage or hematoma. The team:

- identifies the purpose, goals, and scope and defines the target population for this guideline
- analyzes problems with guideline compliance, identifies opportunities for improvement, and communicates best practices to frontline teams
- monitors measures to determine if changes lead to improvement, identifies process and outcome metrics, and tracks performance using these metrics
- determines appropriate facility resources for effective and permanent adoption of practices

MANAGEMENT OF BLOOD LOSS

Interventions include applying pressure to the site and being prepared to return the patient to the operating room:

- Develop a standard set of criteria or early warning signs to trigger notification of the responsible surgeon of possible postoperative bleeding.
- Incorporate all components of the criteria/early warning signs into a tool designed to provide

standardized documentation of all pertinent event details. This tool will provide data to track patient characteristics, processes, and outcomes for continuous quality improvement.
- Establish a policy to empower nurses to rapidly escalate up the chain of authority to reach the responsible surgeon, with a five-minute time limit after the initial page before notifying the next higher level of authority.
- Provide educational sessions to all clinical staff on the pilot units (nurses, residents, attending physicians, other providers, respiratory therapists, patient care technicians, certified nursing assistants, etc.) on the use of the early warning signs criteria, required documentation, and policy for rapid escalation up the chain of authority to notify the responsible surgeon.

Common early warning signs of hemorrhage include, but are not limited to:
- restlessness and anxiety
- frank bleeding and bruising
- tachycardia
- diminished cardiac output and dropping central venous pressure
- reductions in urine output
- swelling and discoloration of the extremities

MEDICATION MANAGEMENT

- Develop a process and protocol for determining if discontinuing antiplatelet or anticoagulant medications before a procedure or surgery is appropriate.
- Select practice recommendations based on individual patient risk factors and current evidence-based guidelines for a particular surgery.
- Obtain a thorough history of medication use before the surgery, specifically addressing the use of over-the-counter (OTC) and prescribed medications.

- Document this information in the patient's medical record to be available to all care providers.

EDUCATIONAL RECOMMENDATIONS

- Provide education on protocols to physicians and other providers, nurses, and all other staff involved in operative and procedural cases and the care of patients postoperatively. Education should occur upon hire, annually, and when this protocol is added to job responsibilities.

EFFECTIVENESS OF ACTION ITEMS

- Track compliance with elements of the established protocol using checklists, appropriate documentation, and so on.
- Evaluate the effectiveness of new processes, determine gaps, modify processes as needed, and reimplement practices.
- Ensure that all personnel follow the protocols and practices developed by the team to prevent postoperative hemorrhage and hematoma, and develop a plan of action for staff who are noncompliant.
- Provide feedback to all stakeholders (physicians and other providers, nursing and ancillary staff, senior medical staff, and executive medical and administrative leadership) on compliance with the process.
- Conduct surveillance and determine the prevalence of postoperative hemorrhage to evaluate the outcomes of new processes.
- Regularly monitor and evaluate performance to sustain improvements achieved.[1]

---

[1] Agency for Healthcare Research and Quality (AHRQ), "PSI 09: Postoperative Hemorrhage or Hematoma," U.S. Department of Health and Human Services (HHS), March 15, 2012. Available online. URL: www.ahrq.gov/sites/default/files/wysiwyg/professionals/systems/hospital/qitoolkit/combined/d4f_combo_psi09-postophemorrhage-bestpractices.pdf. Accessed April 12, 2024.

BLOOD TRANSFUSION

A blood transfusion is a common, safe medical procedure in which healthy donor blood is given to you through an intravenous (IV) line inserted in one of your blood vessels. Blood transfusions replace blood lost through surgery or injury. This treatment also provides blood if your body is not making blood properly on its own.

Four types of blood products may be given through blood transfusions:

- whole blood
- red blood cells (RBCs), which carry oxygen throughout the body
- platelets, which help your blood clot
- plasma, the fluid part of blood

Most of the blood used for transfusions comes from whole blood donations given by volunteer blood donors. Sometimes people have their own blood collected and stored a few weeks before elective surgery in case it is needed.

After a doctor determines that you need a blood transfusion, your blood will be tested to ensure that the blood you are given is a good match. Blood transfusions usually take one to four hours to complete. You will be monitored during and after the procedure.

Blood transfusions are usually very safe because donated blood is carefully tested, handled, and stored. However, there is a small chance that your body may have a mild or even a severe reaction to the donor blood.

Other complications of blood transfusions may include:

- fever
- heart or lung problems
- alloimmunization, when the body's natural defense system attacks donor blood cells
- rare but serious reactions where donated white blood cells (WBCs) attack your body's healthy tissues

Some people also have health problems from getting too much iron after frequent transfusions. There is also a very small chance of getting an infectious disease such as hepatitis B or C or human immunodeficiency virus (HIV) through a blood transfusion. For HIV, that chance is less than one in one million. Scientific research and careful medical controls make the supply of donated blood very safe.[2]

[2] "Treatments for Blood Disorders," National Heart, Lung, and Blood Institute (NHLBI), March 24, 2022. Available online. URL: www.nhlbi.nih.gov/health/blood-bone-marrow-treatments. Accessed April 12, 2024.

Chapter 31 | **Infections and Surgical Complications**

Chapter Contents

IMPORTANCE OF PREVENTING INFECTIONS

You can help protect yourself from infections when you get medical care. This is especially important when you have a medical procedure, such as surgery or dialysis.

STEPS TO PREVENT INFECTIONS DURING MEDICAL PROCEDURES

- Talk with your doctor or nurse about infections.
- Ensure your doctors, nurses, and visitors always wash their hands—and wash your own hands often, too.
- Follow the instructions your doctor gives you for preventing infections after your procedure.

RISK FACTORS FOR INFECTIONS

Germs can spread from one patient to another or from doctors and nurses to patients. You are at higher risk of getting infections from germs if:

- You have surgery, or you get an IV (intravenous) tube, a catheter (tube in your vein or bladder), or a ventilator (breathing tube).
- You are very sick.
- Your doctors, nurses, and visitors do not take steps to prevent infections, such as washing their hands.
- You take unnecessary antibiotics.

The good news is that patients and doctors can work together to prevent the spread of germs and the infections they cause.

TYPES OF INFECTIONS

Health-Care-Associated Infections

Infections caused by visiting a hospital, health clinic, doctor's office, or other health-care facility are called "health-care-associated infections" (HAIs). These infections can lead to sickness and even death. Examples of HAIs include blood infections and urinary tract infections from catheters.

Common Types of Health-Care-Associated Infections

- urinary tract infections (UTIs)
- pneumonia
- blood infections
- methicillin-resistant *Staphylococcus aureus* (MRSA) infections
- surgical site infections
- *C. diff* (*Clostridium difficile*) infections

SIGNS OF INFECTION

Common signs that you may have an infection include:

- fever
- burning or pain below the stomach (the lower abdomen)
- burning or pain when urinating or having to urinate more often than usual
- redness or pain around a catheter or wound
- pus or other liquid coming from the skin
- diarrhea (frequent, watery stool)
- pain that you were not having before

COMMUNICATION WITH HEALTH-CARE PROVIDERS

Preventing Infections through Communication

Before having surgery or getting another type of medical procedure, talk with your doctor or nurse about:

- any medical problems you have, like diabetes, since some medical problems can raise your risk of getting an infection
- what your health-care team will do before the procedure to help prevent an infection, like cleaning the skin with soap
- what you can do to help protect yourself from an infection after the procedure

Start the conversation by saying, "I know how easy it is for people to get infections. I do not want it to happen to me."

Addressing Concerns and Observations

Do not be afraid to speak up and ask questions before or after your procedure. For example, if your bandages are not clean, dry, or attached well, point this out to the doctor or nurse. Your safety is their priority.

After your procedure, pay close attention to changes in your health. If you get home and start to feel sick or notice signs of an infection, call your doctor or nurse right away.

POST-PROCEDURE CARE

Following Instructions to Prevent Infections

It is important to follow all the instructions you get for what to do after a medical procedure, including:

- washing your hands with soap and water often—especially after using the bathroom, before eating, and before touching a wound or catheter
- asking every day if it is time for the catheter to be removed if you have one
- keeping any follow-up appointments

Using Medicines Safely

You may need to take antibiotics or other medicines after a procedure. Be sure to follow the instructions on when, how often, and how long to take them.

If you are taking antibiotics:

- take all doses of the antibiotic unless your doctor tells you to stop
- never share antibiotics with other people
- safely dispose of any antibiotics that you do not use
- tell your doctor or nurse if you start having diarrhea

Call your doctor, nurse, or pharmacist immediately if you have any questions about your medicine—or if you are worried that your medicine is making you feel worse.[1]

TIPS TO AVOID HEALTH-CARE-ASSOCIATED INFECTIONS

Follow these six tips to help you and your loved ones prevent HAIs:

1. **Speak up and ask questions.** Advocate for yourself and your loved ones by talking with the health-care professionals caring for you. When a specific treatment is recommended, such as an IV or urinary catheter, ask why it is needed, what the risks are, and when it can be removed. Write down your questions in advance to help remember details. You should feel empowered to ask questions and share any concerns.
2. **Keep your hands clean.** Make sure that everyone around you, including health-care professionals, caregivers, and visitors, cleans their hands with soap and water or with alcohol-based hand sanitizers when they enter or leave your room and just before touching you or your devices, dressings, or equipment. If you do not see a health-care professional clean their hands, simply remind them to "please clean your hands, thank you." If everyone routinely washed their hands, countless deaths could be prevented.
3. **Be antibiotics aware.** Antibiotics do not treat respiratory infections caused by viruses, like colds, flu, and coronavirus 2019 (COVID-19). Never demand an antibiotic if it is not prescribed. When antibiotics are unnecessary, they will not help you, and the side effects can be harmful. Even when needed, antibiotics can still cause side effects and contribute to antimicrobial resistance. Talk with a health-care professional about the best treatment for your illness.

---

[1] Office of Disease Prevention and Health Promotion (ODPHP), "Prevent Infections When You Get Medical Care," U.S. Department of Health and Human Services (HHS), March 30, 2023. https://health.gov/myhealthfinder/healthy-living/safety/prevent-infections-when-you-get-medical-care#take-action-tab. Accessed July 17, 2024.

4. **Recognize the signs and symptoms of an infection.** Learn how to recognize early symptoms of an infection, such as a fever. If you have recently had surgery, look out for redness, pain, or drainage where the incision was made in your skin without touching the site directly. Never touch IV lines. Keep cuts and wounds clean and covered until healed. If you have a urinary catheter, look for signs of a urinary infection, such as pain or burning when urinating. Talk with a health-care professional about what signs and symptoms you should look for and what to do to ensure prompt and proper treatment if you do get an infection. If an infection is not stopped, it can cause sepsis, a life-threatening medical emergency. Health-care professionals should immediately evaluate and treat people who might have sepsis.
5. **Stay up-to-date on all recommended vaccines.** Staying up-to-date on all recommended vaccines can help you stay healthy, avoiding the need for health care in the first place. Everyone ages six months and older should get an annual flu vaccine and stay up-to-date with their COVID-19 vaccines. Talk with a health-care professional about other vaccines you may need.
6. **Do not be a dreaded spreader.** Do not share your germs when visiting someone in a hospital, nursing home, or other health-care facility. Do not visit a health-care facility if you do not feel well. Wash your hands often. Stay home when sick and use precautions, such as wearing a mask where and when required. Masks can help reduce the spread of some germs.

All of us—patients, caregivers, loved ones, and health-care professionals—play a role in preventing HAIs. Follow these tips to help protect yourself and those you love.[2]

---

[2] "Six Tips for Patients to Avoid Healthcare-Associated Infections," Centers for Disease Control and Prevention (CDC), April 15, 2024. https://blogs.cdc.gov/safehealthcare/6-tips-for-patients-to-avoid-healthcare-associated-infections. Accessed July 17, 2024.

Section 31.2 | Preventing and Managing Postoperative Infections and Sepsis

SURGICAL SITE INFECTIONS

Overview

A surgical site infection (SSI) is a type of health-care-associated infection (HAI). It occurs in the part of the body where surgery took place.

Types of Surgical Site Infections

Surgical site infections can occur in:

- skin
- tissue
- organs
- implanted material, such as a hip replacement

Signs and Symptoms

- redness and pain around the area where you had surgery
- cloudy fluid draining from your surgical wound
- fever
- other signs and symptoms may also occur

Reducing the Risk of Surgical Site Infections

BEFORE SURGERY

- **Tell your health-care provider about other medical problems you may have.** Health issues such as allergies, diabetes, and obesity could affect your surgery and your treatment.
- **Quit smoking.** Patients who smoke get more infections. Talk to your health-care provider about how you can quit before your surgery.
- **Do not shave near where you will have surgery.** Shaving with a razor can irritate your skin and make it easier to develop an infection.

AT THE TIME OF SURGERY

- **Speak up if someone tries to shave you with a razor in the area where you will have surgery**. Ask why you need to be shaved and talk with your surgeon if you have any concerns.

AFTER SURGERY

- If you do not see your health-care provider clean their hands, please ask them to do so.
- Family and friends should not touch the surgical wound or dressings.
- Family and friends should clean their hands with soap and water or an alcohol-based hand rub before and after visiting you. If you do not see them clean their hands, ask them to do so.
- Always clean your hands before and after caring for your wound.

BEFORE YOU LEAVE THE HOSPITAL

- Make sure you understand how to care for your wound.
- Ensure you know who to contact if you have questions or problems.

ONCE YOU ARE HOME

- If you have any symptoms of an infection, such as redness and pain at the surgery site, drainage, or fever, call your health-care provider immediately.
- Health-care providers should always follow core infection control practices and SSI prevention guidelines to reduce the risk of spreading germs to patients.

Treatment and Recovery

Treatment generally includes antibiotics, but the type of treatment depends on the germ causing the infection. Sometimes, patients need another surgery to treat SSIs.[1]

[1] "Surgical Site Infection Basics," Centers for Disease Control and Prevention (CDC), April 11, 2024. Available online. URL: www.cdc.gov/surgical-site-infections/about. Accessed July 16, 2024.

SEPSIS

Sepsis is the body's extreme response to an infection, a life-threatening medical emergency. Without prompt treatment, sepsis can lead to tissue damage, organ failure, and death.

Causes of Sepsis

Sepsis occurs when an infection you already have triggers a chain reaction throughout your body. Bacterial infections are the most common cause, but other infections can also cause sepsis. Common sources of infections leading to sepsis include the lungs, stomach, kidneys, or bladder. Sepsis can start with a small cut that gets infected or with an infection after surgery. Sometimes, sepsis occurs in people who did not know they had an infection.

Risk Factors for Sepsis

Anyone with an infection can get sepsis, but certain people are more likely to develop it:

- adults 65 or older
- people with chronic conditions, such as diabetes, lung disease, cancer, and kidney disease
- people with weakened immune systems
- pregnant women
- children younger than one

Symptoms of Sepsis

- rapid breathing and heart rate
- shortness of breath
- confusion or disorientation
- extreme pain or discomfort
- fever, shivering, or feeling very cold
- clammy or sweaty skin

Complications of Sepsis

Severe cases of sepsis can lead to septic shock, where blood pressure drops to a dangerous level, and multiple organs can fail.

Diagnosis of Sepsis

To diagnose sepsis, your health-care provider will:

- take your medical history and ask about your symptoms
- perform a physical exam, including checking vital signs (temperature, blood pressure, heart rate, and breathing)
- likely order lab tests to check for signs of infection or organ damage
- possibly order imaging tests, such as an x-ray or CT scan, to find the infection's location

Since many signs and symptoms of sepsis can also be caused by other medical conditions, diagnosing sepsis in its early stages can be challenging.

Treatments for Sepsis

Prompt treatment for sepsis usually includes:

- antibiotics
- maintaining blood flow to organs, which may involve getting oxygen and intravenous (IV) fluids
- treating the source of the infection
- medications to increase blood pressure if needed

In serious cases, treatments may include kidney dialysis or a breathing tube. Some people might need surgery to remove tissue damaged by the infection.

Prevention of Sepsis

To prevent sepsis, try to prevent infections by:

- taking good care of any chronic health conditions
- getting recommended vaccines
- practicing good hygiene, such as handwashing
- keeping cuts clean and covered until healed[2]

[2] MedlinePlus, "Sepsis," National Institutes of Health (NIH), November 13, 2023. Available online. URL: https://medlineplus.gov/sepsis.html. Accessed April 8, 2024.

Section 31.3 | Central Line-Associated Bloodstream Infections

OVERVIEW

Central line-associated bloodstream infections (CLABSIs) result in thousands of deaths each year and billions of dollars in added costs to the U.S. health-care system—but they are preventable.

A central line (or central venous catheter) is a tube that health-care providers often place in a large vein in the neck, chest, or groin to give medication or fluids or to collect blood for medical tests. Central lines are different from peripheral intravenous (IV) catheters (shorter IV catheters placed in the hand, arm, or foot for vein access); central lines access a major vein close to the heart, can remain in place for weeks or months, and are much more likely to be a source of serious infection. Central lines are commonly used in intensive care units.

Health-care providers may insert central lines to:

- administer medicines for treatment of pain, infection, or other medical issues (e.g., cancer or heart problems)
- provide fluids or nutrition
- conduct certain medical tests

TYPES OF CENTRAL LINES

Peripherally Inserted Central Catheter

- placed into a vein in the arm

Tunneled Catheter

- passed under the skin and placed into a vein in the chest or neck
- providers can insert medicine directly into the catheter

Implanted Port

- surgically placed under the skin
- providers insert medicines using a needle placed through the skin into the catheter

- not as visible as a tunneled catheter, requires less daily care, and does not interfere with regular activities as much as a PICC line or tunneled catheter

Health-care providers use the type of central line that is best for each patient's care.

SIGNS AND SYMPTOMS

People with CLABSIs may experience:

- fever
- red skin and soreness around the central line

CAUSES

Central line-associated bloodstream infections occur when germs (usually bacteria or fungi) enter the bloodstream through the central line.

PREVENTION

Health-care providers should follow recommended infection control guidelines to reduce the risk of CLABSIs.

Patients should:

- **Speak up**. Talk to your health-care providers about any questions or worries. Ask what they are doing to protect you.
- **Discuss options**. Ask a health-care provider about your options and the pros and cons of a central line if needed. If so, ask them to help you understand its need and how long it will be in place.
- **Avoid touching the tubing**. Avoid touching the tubing and where it exits the skin as much as possible.

By following these guidelines and maintaining strict hygiene practices, health-care providers and patients can significantly reduce the risk of CLABSIs.[1]

[1] "Central Line-Associated Bloodstream Infection (CLABSI) Basics," Centers for Disease Control and Prevention (CDC), February 21, 2024. Available online. URL: www.cdc.gov/clabsi/about/index.html. Accessed July 16, 2024.

Section 31.4 | Catheter-Associated Urinary Tract Infections

OVERVIEW

A catheter-associated urinary tract infection (CAUTI) occurs when germs enter the urinary tract through a urinary catheter and cause infection. It is one of the most common health-care-associated infections (HAIs), but is preventable and treatable.

QUICK FACTS

- Catheter-associated urinary tract infections are one of the most common HAIs.
- About 75 percent of urinary tract infections (UTIs) developed in hospitals are associated with a urinary catheter.
- 15–25 percent of hospitalized patients use urinary catheters.
- CAUTIs are associated with increased morbidity, mortality, health-care costs, and length of stay.

SIGNS AND SYMPTOMS

People with CAUTIs may experience:

- burning or pain in the lower abdomen (below the stomach)
- fever
- burning while urinating
- increased frequency of urination

RISK FACTORS

The most important risk factor for developing a CAUTI is prolonged use of a urinary catheter.

CAUSES

A CAUTI occurs when germs (usually bacteria) enter the body through a urinary catheter and cause infection. The infection can occur in any part of the urinary tract, including the kidneys, ureters, bladder, and urethra.

REDUCING RISK

Patients with a urinary catheter should:

- understand why they need the catheter and frequently ask health-care providers if the catheter is still necessary
- if the patient has a long-term catheter, they must clean their hands before and after touching the catheter
- check the position of the urine bag; it should always be below the level of the bladder

Patients with a urinary catheter should not:

- tug or pull on the tubing
- twist or kink the catheter tubing

Health-care workers and facilities can prevent CAUTIs and protect patients with proper infection control processes.

TYPES OF CATHETERS

Indwelling Urinary Catheter

- A drainage tube is inserted into the bladder through the urethra, left in place, and connected to a closed collection system.

Intermittent ("In-and-Out") Catheterization

- Brief insertion of a catheter into the bladder through the urethra to drain urine, followed by removal.

External Catheter

- A urine containment device attached to a urinary drainage bag that fits over or adheres to the genitalia. The most commonly used external catheter is a soft, flexible sheath that fits over the penis (also known as a "condom" catheter).

Suprapubic Catheter

- Surgically inserted into the bladder through an incision in the lower abdomen.

TREATMENT AND RECOVERY

Most CAUTIs can be treated with antibiotics and/or catheter removal or change. The health-care provider will determine the best treatment for each patient.

By following these guidelines and maintaining strict hygiene practices, health-care providers and patients can significantly reduce the risk of CAUTIs and promote a safer recovery environment.[1]

Section 31.5 | **Ventilator-Associated Pneumonia**

OVERVIEW

Ventilator-associated pneumonia (VAP) is a type of health-care-associated infection (HAI). It is a lung infection that develops in a person who is on a ventilator.

CAUSES

Ventilator-associated pneumonia occurs when bacteria enter a patient's lungs and cause an infection.

REDUCING RISK

To minimize the risk of VAP, patients and health-care providers should consider the following:

- **Quit smoking**. Patients who smoke are more prone to infections. Seek information about quitting before surgery.
- **Hand hygiene**. Ensure health-care providers clean their hands before touching the patient or equipment.

[1] "Catheter-Associated Urinary Tract Infection Basics," Centers for Disease Control and Prevention (CDC), April 15, 2024. Available online. URL: www.cdc.gov/uti/about/cauti-basics.html. Accessed July 16, 2024.

- **Bed positioning.** Ask about raising the head of the bed to reduce the risk of aspiration.
- **Weaning from ventilator.** Inquire when the patient can attempt breathing without the ventilator.
- **Oral care.** Ask how often health-care providers clean the patient's mouth to prevent infection.

Health-care providers should always follow core infection prevention and control practices to reduce the risk of spreading germs to patients. Acute care hospitals should implement strategies to prevent VAP.

TREATMENT AND RECOVERY

Treatment for VAP generally includes antibiotics. The specific type of antibiotic depends on the bacteria causing the infection. The health-care provider will determine which antibiotic is best for each patient.

By following these guidelines and maintaining strict hygiene practices, health-care providers and patients can significantly reduce the risk of VAP and promote a safer recovery environment.[1]

Section 31.6 | Methicillin-Resistant *Staphylococcus aureus* Infections

OVERVIEW

Staphylococcus aureus (staph) is a very common germ. About one out of every three people have the germ on their skin or in their nose. This germ does not cause problems for most people.

Methicillin-resistant *Staphylococcus aureus* (MRSA) is a type of staph that can resist several antibiotics. Anyone can get a MRSA infection or carry MRSA. The risk increases for people with hospitalizations

[1] "Ventilator-Associated Pneumonia Basics," Centers for Disease Control and Prevention (CDC), January 22, 2024. Available online. URL: www.cdc.gov/ventilator-associated-pneumonia/about. Accessed July 16, 2024.

or nursing home stays, skin-to-skin contact with others (such as in contact sports), and exposure to crowded and unhygienic places.

SIGNS AND SYMPTOMS *STAPHYLOCOCCUS AUREUS* INFECTION

The symptoms of an *S. aureus* infection, including MRSA, depend on the part of the infected body. Broken skin, such as scrapes or cuts, is often the site of a MRSA infection. Most *S. aureus* skin infections, including MRSA, appear as a bump or infected area on the skin that might be:

- red
- swollen
- painful
- warm to the touch
- full of pus or other drainage
- accompanied by a fever

You cannot tell by looking at the skin if it is a MRSA infection. People sometimes confuse some MRSA skin infections with a spider bite. However, unless you actually see the spider, the irritation is likely not a spider bite.

If you or someone in your family experiences the signs and symptoms of MRSA infection:

- Contact your health-care provider, especially if the symptoms include a fever or do not improve within 48 hours.
- Do not pick at or pop the bump or sore.
- Cover the area with clean, dry bandages until you can see a health-care provider.
- Clean your hands often.

COMPLICATIONS OF METHICILLIN-RESISTANT *STAPHYLOCOCCUS AUREUS* INFECTIONS

Methicillin-resistant *Staphylococcus aureus* infections can cause serious problems in and outside health-care settings, including:

- pneumonia (lung infections)
- bloodstream infections

- surgical site infections
- sepsis, the body's extreme response to an infection (if left untreated)
- death (if left untreated)

WHO IS AT RISK?

Although anyone can get MRSA, some groups have a higher risk:

- people who receive inpatient medical care
- people who have surgery or medical devices inserted in their body
- people who inject drugs
- athletes
- daycare and school students
- military personnel in barracks

HOW IT SPREADS

Methicillin-resistant *Staphylococcus aureus* spreads in the community through contact with infected people, wounds, or objects that have touched infected skin and are carrying the bacteria. Some people who carry MRSA can go on to get an MRSA infection.

PREVENTION OF METHICILLIN-RESISTANT *STAPHYLOCOCCUS AUREUS* INFECTIONS

Maintaining good hygiene and taking precautions in environments with a higher risk of MRSA infections can reduce your risk of infection and help prevent its spread.

DIAGNOSIS OF METHICILLIN-RESISTANT *STAPHYLOCOCCUS AUREUS* INFECTIONS

A health-care provider must send a clinical specimen to a laboratory to determine if MRSA is the cause of an infection.

TREATMENT AND RECOVERY

Health-care providers often prescribe antibiotics to treat MRSA infections. Some types of *S. aureus* infections need surgery to drain infected areas. Your health-care provider will determine which treatments are best for you. While MRSA can resist several antibiotics, meaning these drugs cannot cure the infections, antibiotics are available to treat MRSA infections.[1]

[1] "Methicillin-Resistant *Staphylococcus aureus* (MRSA) Basics," Centers for Disease Control and Prevention (CDC), April 11, 2024. Available online. URL: www.cdc.gov/mrsa/about. Accessed July 16, 2024.

Chapter 32 | **Other Surgical Complications**

Chapter Contents

WHAT ARE ABDOMINAL ADHESIONS?

Abdominal adhesions are bands of scar-like tissue that form inside the abdomen. These bands can form between two or more organs or between organs and the abdominal wall. Normally, the surfaces of organs and the abdominal wall do not stick together when you move. However, abdominal adhesions may cause these surfaces to adhere or stick together. This can lead to kinking, twisting, pulling, or compressing the intestines and other organs, causing symptoms and complications such as intestinal obstruction or blockage.

HOW COMMON ARE ABDOMINAL ADHESIONS?

Abdominal adhesions are common and often develop after abdominal surgery. Surgeons enter a patient's abdomen through an incision during abdominal surgery, which may be laparoscopic or open. In laparoscopic surgery, small cuts are made in the abdomen, and special tools are inserted to view, remove, or repair organs and tissues. In open surgery, a larger cut is made to open the abdomen. More than 9 out of every 10 people who have surgery that opens the abdomen develop abdominal adhesions. However, a majority of these people do not develop symptoms or complications. Abdominal adhesions are less common after laparoscopic surgery than after open surgery.

WHAT CAUSES ABDOMINAL ADHESIONS?

Abdominal surgery is the most common cause of abdominal adhesions. Adhesions caused by surgery are more likely to cause symptoms and complications than those related to other causes. Symptoms and complications may start any time after surgery, even many years later. Conditions that involve inflammation or infection in the abdomen may also cause adhesions. These conditions include Crohn's disease, diverticular disease, endometriosis, pelvic inflammatory disease (PID), and peritonitis. Other causes include long-term peritoneal dialysis to treat kidney failure and radiation therapy to treat cancer. In some cases, abdominal adhesions are present at birth.

WHO IS MORE LIKELY TO HAVE ABDOMINAL ADHESIONS?

People who have had abdominal surgery are more likely to have abdominal adhesions. Among those who have had abdominal surgery, adhesions and related complications are more common in people who:

- had emergency abdominal surgery
- had pelvic surgery or surgery involving the lower digestive tract, including the colon and rectum

WHAT ARE THE SYMPTOMS OF ABDOMINAL ADHESIONS?

In many cases, abdominal adhesions do not cause symptoms. If they do, chronic abdominal pain is the most common symptom. Abdominal adhesions may cause intestinal obstruction, which can be life-threatening. Symptoms of intestinal obstruction may include:

- abdominal pain
- bloating
- constipation
- not passing gas
- nausea
- vomiting

If intestinal obstruction cuts off blood flow to the blocked part of the intestines or leads to peritonitis, additional symptoms, such as a fast heart rate or fever, may develop.

HOW DO DOCTORS DIAGNOSE ABDOMINAL ADHESIONS?

Doctors diagnose abdominal adhesions using medical history, physical exams, blood tests, imaging tests, and, in some cases, surgery.

Medical History

A doctor will ask about your symptoms and medical history, including your history of abdominal surgery or other conditions that may cause abdominal adhesions. They will also ask about other diseases and disorders that may cause similar symptoms.

Physical Exam

During a physical exam, the doctor may tap on your abdomen to check for tenderness or pain and use a stethoscope to listen to sounds in your abdomen.

Blood Tests

A health-care professional will take blood samples and send them to a lab. While blood tests cannot diagnose abdominal adhesions, they can help rule out other health problems that could be causing your symptoms. If you have signs of an intestinal obstruction, blood tests can help determine its severity.

Imaging Tests

Imaging tests most often cannot show abdominal adhesions. However, they can help diagnose intestinal obstruction caused by adhesions and rule out other problems. Imaging tests may include:

- **Computed tomography (CT)**. Uses x-rays and computer technology to create images. A CT scan may help diagnose intestinal obstruction and find its location, cause, and severity.
- **X-rays**. Use a small amount of radiation to create pictures of the inside of the body.
- **X-rays with water-soluble contrast medium**. This special liquid makes the digestive tract more visible on x-rays. It can help doctors determine if surgery is needed and may also help relieve the obstruction.
- **Lower gastrointestinal (GI) series**. Uses x-rays to view the large intestine.

Surgery

In some cases, doctors may recommend surgery to look inside the abdomen and check for adhesions or other problems. Surgeons may check for abdominal adhesions with laparoscopic or open surgery and may be able to treat the problem during the procedure.

HOW DO DOCTORS TREAT ABDOMINAL ADHESIONS?

If abdominal adhesions do not cause symptoms or complications, they typically do not need treatment. If they do cause symptoms or complications, doctors can release the adhesions with laparoscopic or open surgery. However, surgery to treat adhesions may cause new adhesions to form. If you have abdominal adhesions, talk with your doctor about the possible benefits and risks of surgery.

If adhesions cause an intestinal obstruction, immediate hospital treatment is necessary. Doctors will examine you and may order tests to determine if emergency surgery is needed. If so, surgeons will release the adhesions, relieving the obstruction. If emergency surgery is not needed, doctors may try to treat the obstruction without surgery by providing intravenous (IV) fluids and inserting a tube through your nose into your stomach to remove the contents of your digestive tract above the obstruction. If the obstruction does not resolve, surgery will be performed.

WHAT ARE THE COMPLICATIONS OF ABDOMINAL ADHESIONS?

Intestinal Obstruction

Intestinal obstruction is the partial or complete blockage of the movement of food, fluids, air, or stool through the intestines. Abdominal adhesions are the most common cause of small intestine obstruction. This condition may lead to:

- lack of blood flow to the blocked part of the intestine and death of the blood-starved intestinal tissues
- peritonitis, an infection of the lining of the abdominal cavity

Intestinal obstruction can be life-threatening. People with symptoms of a complete blockage—such as abdominal pain and inability to pass fluids, stool, or gas—should seek medical attention immediately.

Female Infertility

In women, abdominal adhesions in the pelvis or inside the uterus can compress or block parts of the reproductive system and cause infertility.

CAN ABDOMINAL ADHESIONS BE PREVENTED?

Surgeons take steps to lower the chance of developing abdominal adhesions and related complications after surgery. For example, they may:

- recommend laparoscopic surgery, if possible, instead of open surgery
- handle tissues gently to prevent damage
- take steps to keep foreign materials out of the abdomen, such as using powder-free gloves and lint-free tools
- cover damaged tissues inside the abdomen with a special film-like barrier at the end of surgery (This barrier keeps tissues separated while they heal and is then absorbed by the body.)[1]

Section 32.2 | **Health-Care-Associated Venous Thromboembolism**

WHAT IS HEALTH-CARE-ASSOCIATED VENOUS THROMBOEMBOLISM?

People who are currently or recently hospitalized or recovering from surgery are at increased risk of developing serious and potentially deadly blood clots, known as "venous thromboembolism" (VTE). A blood clot that occurs as a result of hospitalization, surgery, or other health-care treatment or procedure is called "health-care-associated venous thromboembolism" (HA-VTE).

[1] "Abdominal Adhesions," National Institute of Diabetes and Digestive and Kidney Diseases (NIDDK), June 2019. Available online. URL: www.niddk.nih.gov/health-information/digestive-diseases/abdominal-adhesions. Accessed April 10, 2024.

WHO IS AT RISK FOR HEALTH-CARE-ASSOCIATED VENOUS THROMBOEMBOLISM?

Several specific health-care-associated factors increase the risk of developing deep vein thrombosis (DVT) or pulmonary embolism (PE). These include:

- injury to a vein, often caused by:
  - fractures
  - severe muscle injury
  - major surgery (particularly involving the abdomen, pelvis, hip, or legs)
- slow blood flow, often caused by:
  - confinement to bed
  - limited movement (e.g., a cast on a leg to help heal an injured bone)
- other health-care-associated factors:
  - a catheter located in a central vein
- certain factors put you at even greater risk of HA-VTE when combined with hospitalization, surgery, and/or immobility (limited movement):
  - a previous blood clot
  - an inherited clotting disorder
  - a family history of blood clots
  - overweight or obesity
  - age 55 or older
  - taking hormonal medications
  - currently or recently pregnant (within 3 months of giving birth)
  - currently being treated for cancer
  - having other medical conditions like AIDS, anemia, arthritis, diabetes, high blood pressure, or heart disease

TIMES OF INCREASED RISK

Recent studies have found:

- Among patients who developed a blood clot after surgery, 40 percent occurred while they were still in the hospital, while 60 percent occurred up to 90 days after leaving the hospital.

- More than half of blood clots first identified in an outpatient setting are directly linked to a recent hospitalization or surgery.
- Most health-care providers do not reassess the risk of VTE at hospital discharge.

WHY IS HEALTH-CARE-ASSOCIATED VENOUS THROMBOEMBOLISM A PUBLIC HEALTH PROBLEM?

Although anyone can develop a blood clot, more than a third of blood clots diagnosed each year are related to a recent hospitalization, and most of these do not occur until after discharge.

- VTE is a leading cause of preventable hospital death in the United States.
- VTE is the fifth most frequent reason for unplanned hospital readmissions after surgery and the third most frequent among patients undergoing total hip or knee joint replacement.
- Patients with HA-VTE are three times more likely to be readmitted to the hospital than patients without HA-VTE.
- As many as 70 percent of cases of HA-VTE are preventable through measures such as using blood-thinning medications called "anticoagulants," which help prevent blood from clotting, or using compression stockings. Yet fewer than half of hospital patients receive these measures.

PROTECTING YOURSELF FROM BLOOD CLOTS AFTER HOSPITALIZATION OR SURGERY

Know the signs and symptoms of blood clots. Discuss your risks with your health-care providers.

A blood clot occurring in the legs or arms is called "deep vein thrombosis" (DVT). Signs and symptoms of a DVT include:

- swelling of the affected limb
- pain or tenderness not caused by injury
- skin that is warm to the touch, red, or discolored

If you have the signs or symptoms of a DVT, alert your health-care provider as soon as possible.

A blood clot in the legs or arms can break off and travel to the lungs. This is called a "pulmonary embolism" (PE) and can be life-threatening. Signs and symptoms of PE include:

- difficulty breathing
- chest pain that usually worsens with a deep breath or cough
- cough or coughing up blood
- faster than normal or irregular heartbeat

Seek immediate medical attention if you experience any signs or symptoms of a possible PE.

Talk with your health-care providers about factors that might increase your risk for a blood clot. Let them know if you or anyone in your family has ever had a blood clot.[1]

Section 32.3 | **Postlumbar Puncture Headache**

WHAT IS LUMBAR PUNCTURE?

A lumbar puncture (LP) is an outpatient procedure where a small needle is inserted between the vertebrae (spinal bones) of the lower back at a level below the spinal cord to obtain a small amount of cerebrospinal fluid (CSF). It is sometimes referred to as a "spinal tap."

WHAT IS THE PURPOSE OF A LUMBAR PUNCTURE?

The purpose of obtaining spinal fluid is to learn as much as possible about the proteins and other chemical changes that may occur in individuals with neurological conditions, such as Parkinson disease

[1] "Understanding Your Risk for Healthcare-Associated VTE (Blood Clots)," Centers for Disease Control and Prevention (CDC), May 15, 2024. Available online. URL: www.cdc.gov/blood-clots/risk-factors/ha-vte.html. Accessed July 17, 2024.

(PD) and Lewy body dementia (LBD). Spinal fluid is useful because it bathes the brain and spinal cord, making it the best source of information about neurochemical changes that may be occurring in the brain. Because many proteins do not cross from the spinal fluid into the bloodstream, spinal fluid is sometimes the only way to see that something is wrong with the brain. Scientists predict that proteins in the spinal fluid could be promising biomarkers of PD and related conditions. Being able to measure changes in specific proteins or neurochemicals in spinal fluid may provide a way to predict disease progression, evaluate why symptoms vary from person to person, and monitor if new treatments can slow progression of the disease.

WHAT HAPPENS DURING THE PROCEDURE?

The lumbar puncture can be done in two positions: while you lie curled up on one side with knees close to the chest, or while you lean forward over a table while seated. The doctor will locate a puncture site in the lower back, between two vertebrae, then clean the area and inject a local anesthetic. You may feel a slight stinging sensation from this injection. Once the anesthetic has taken effect, the doctor will insert a special needle into the spinal sac and collect a small amount of fluid (usually about three teaspoons) for testing. This spinal fluid is normally replenished within one hour. Sometimes, a special x-ray or ultrasound may be used to help the doctor guide the needle into the right place. The entire procedure takes about 45 minutes.

IS A LUMBAR PUNCTURE PAINFUL?

There are two parts in the beginning of the LP procedure that may cause some discomfort. First, during the administration of an anesthetic, you may feel a few seconds of stinging or burning when it is injected. Second, you may also feel a pressure sensation when the needle is inserted, and there is usually some brief pain when the needle goes through the tissue surrounding the spinal cord. Overall, discomfort throughout the entire procedure is minimal to moderate.

WHAT ARE THE RISKS OF LUMBAR PUNCTURE?

There is a small chance of developing a headache after the procedure. This usually gets better with rest and drinking plenty of fluids. Rarely, the headache may continue for more than 24 hours after the procedure and require additional treatment. There is no risk of paralysis. LPs are typically performed using a special needle designed for this procedure. LP needles have improved over time and are now smaller, causing less pain at the site where the needle goes in and are less likely to cause headache after the LP. When performed by an experienced doctor, an LP is safe and involves minimal discomfort.[1]

WHAT IS THE CURE FOR POSTLUMBAR PUNCTURE HEADACHE?

Since the headache occurs only when the individual stands up, the cure is to lie down until the headache runs its course—anywhere from a few hours to several days. Severe postdural headaches may be treated by injecting a small amount of the individual's own blood into the low back to stop the leak (called an "epidural blood patch"). Occasionally, spinal fluid leaks spontaneously, causing this "low-pressure headache."[2]

Section 32.4 | **Cardiogenic Shock**

WHAT IS CARDIOGENIC SHOCK?

Cardiogenic shock, or cardiac shock, occurs when the heart cannot pump enough blood and oxygen to the brain and other vital organs. This life-threatening emergency is treatable if diagnosed promptly, making it crucial to recognize the warning signs. Without sufficient oxygen-rich blood reaching vital organs, blood pressure drops, and the pulse slows, leading to symptoms such as confusion, sweating, and rapid breathing. Unconsciousness may also occur.

---

[1] "Facts about Lumbar Puncture," National Institute of Neurological Disorders and Stroke (NINDS), August 16, 2018. Available online. URL: https://pdbp.ninds.nih.gov/facts-about-LP. Accessed July 17, 2024.

[2] "Headache," National Institute of Neurological Disorders and Stroke (NINDS), November 28, 2023. Available online. URL: www.ninds.nih.gov/health-information/disorders/headache. Accessed July 17, 2024.

CAUSES OF CARDIOGENIC SHOCK

A heart attack is the most common cause of cardiogenic shock. Other health issues, including heart failure, chest injuries, and blood clots in the lungs, can also lead to this condition.

Heart Attack and Other Heart Problems

Cardiogenic shock usually develops quickly following a heart attack. Other heart conditions, such as heart failure or arrhythmia, can impede the heart's ability to deliver oxygen-rich blood to the organs, resulting in cardiogenic shock.

Heart Procedures

Certain heart procedures, such as cardiac catheterization, may occasionally cause cardiogenic shock due to injury to the heart or arrhythmias.

Problems outside the Heart

Cardiogenic shock can be caused by issues outside the heart, such as fluid buildup in the chest, internal bleeding, or pulmonary embolism (a blood clot in a lung artery). Trauma or injury to the chest can damage the heart, reducing its ability to pump blood effectively.

Medicines

Rarely, some medicines can cause cardiogenic shock if taken in excessive doses or if the heart is weakened after a heart attack or other heart problem. Medicines like beta-blockers or calcium channel blockers, used to treat high blood pressure (HBP), can sometimes lead to this condition.

RISK FACTORS FOR CARDIOGENIC SHOCK

Certain factors may increase the risk for cardiogenic shock:

- age 75 or older
- Asian Americans and Pacific Islanders (less likely to receive emergency treatment compared to whites)

- more common in women than men (Women are also less likely to receive emergency treatment.)
- heart and blood vessel problems, such as coronary heart disease, heart failure, and HBP
- diabetes and prediabetes
- overweight and obesity
- past coronary artery bypass grafting (CABG)
- pneumothorax (collapsed lung)
- sepsis (life-threatening inflammatory response to infection)

SYMPTOMS OF CARDIOGENIC SHOCK

Symptoms vary depending on the severity and speed of blood pressure drop. Common signs include:

- low blood pressure (feeling dizzy, confused, or nauseous)
- weak or irregular pulse

Additional symptoms may include:

- rapid or severe shortness of breath
- bulging neck vein
- clammy skin
- cold hands and feet
- fever
- loss of consciousness
- swelling of feet
- decreased urination
- cardiac arrest

DIAGNOSIS OF CARDIOGENIC SHOCK

To diagnose cardiogenic shock, doctors use a combination of medical history, physical exams, and diagnostic tests.

Medical History

Doctors will inquire about symptoms and history of heart attacks or other relevant conditions.

Physical Exam
Doctors check for cold extremities, weak pulse, abnormal heart and lung sounds, urine output, and low blood pressure.

Diagnostic Tests and Procedures
Common tests include:
- chest x-ray
- coronary angiography
- echocardiography
- electrocardiogram (ECG or EKG)
- blood gas tests
- blood tests for organ function and lactic acid levels
- other heart imaging tests

TREATMENT FOR CARDIOGENIC SHOCK
Cardiogenic shock is life-threatening but treatable if addressed promptly. Hospital treatment may include medications, procedures to restore blood flow, and emergency interventions to stabilize the patient.

Medicines
- antiarrhythmia medicines
- blood thinners or antiplatelet medicines
- vasopressors and inotropes (e.g., norepinephrine, dobutamine)

Procedures
- coronary artery bypass grafting (CABG)
- percutaneous coronary intervention (PCI)

Medical Devices
- extracorporeal membrane oxygenation (ECMO)
- intra-aortic balloon pump (IABP)
- percutaneous circulatory assist devices (PCADs), including ventricular assist devices (VADs)

RECOVERY FROM CARDIOGENIC SHOCK

Following treatment, adopting healthy lifestyle changes is essential to prevent recurrence.

Monitor Your Condition

- Have regular follow-ups to monitor health and any medical devices.

Adopt Healthy Lifestyle Changes

- heart-healthy eating (DASH eating plan)
- regular physical activity
- maintaining a healthy weight
- managing stress
- quitting smoking (National Cancer Institute's Smoking Quitline: 877-448-7848)

Cardiac Rehabilitation

- Adopt exercise-based cardiac rehabilitation to manage symptoms and reduce future risks.

Prevent a Repeat Event

- Managing health conditions, such as diabetes and high cholesterol, is crucial to preventing another event.

Take Care of Your Mental Health

- Seek professional counseling, join support groups, and communicate with family and friends about your needs.

Learn the Warning Signs of Serious Complications

- Recognize symptoms of brain injury, heart attack, kidney failure, liver damage, and stroke.

WARNING SIGNS OF COMPLICATIONS

Brain Injury

- Symptoms include poor judgment, memory loss, and decreased coordination.

Heart Attack

- Symptoms include chest pain, discomfort, shortness of breath, nausea, and pain in the back, shoulders, or jaw.

Kidney Failure

- Regular testing of kidney function may be necessary.

Liver Damage

- Symptoms include hypoxic hepatitis or liver failure.

Stroke

If you think someone may be having a stroke, act F.A.S.T. and perform the following simple test.

- **F—Face**. Ask the person to smile. Does one side of the face droop?
- **A—Arms**. Ask the person to raise both arms. Does one arm drift downward?
- **S—Speech**. Ask the person to repeat a simple phrase. Is their speech slurred or strange?
- **T—Time**. If you observe any of these signs, call 911 right away. Early treatment is essential.

Understanding cardiogenic shock, recognizing its symptoms, and following preventive measures can significantly improve outcomes and reduce the risk of recurrence.[1]

[1] "Cardiogenic Shock," National Heart, Lung, and Blood Institute (NHLBI), March 24, 2022. Available online. URL: www.nhlbi.nih.gov/health/cardiogenic-shock. Accessed July 17, 2024.

Part 5 | Recovery and Rehabilitation after Surgery

Chapter 33 | Prehabilitation and Rehabilitation for Total Joint Replacement

OSTEOARTHRITIS AND JOINT REPLACEMENT

Osteoarthritis (OA) is a leading cause of joint disability in the United States. Approximately 54 million people (23% of adults) have OA, and of these, 24 million are limited in their daily activities due to OA. Total joint replacement (TJR)—including total knee arthroplasty (TKA) and total hip arthroplasty (THA)—has been one of the most successful therapies in managing pain and dysfunction of hip and knee joints for end-stage arthritis. Patients who have undergone a TKA or THA experience reduced pain and improved function and quality of life (QOL). As the prevalence of OA has increased, the number of TKAs and THAs has correspondingly increased, making them the most common inpatient surgical procedures covered by Medicare. In 2014, an estimated 680,150 patients in the United States underwent a TKA, and 370,770 underwent a THA. By 2030, it is expected that 1.26 million patients will undergo a TKA annually (an 85% increase from 2014), and 635,000 will undergo a THA (a 71% increase).

POST-SURGERY OUTCOMES AND CHALLENGES

While most patients experience improvements in pain after TJR, deficits in functional performance and strength commonly persist one year after surgery. Full recovery of muscle strength and physical function to a normal level is rare. Additionally, some patients have balance and movement control deficits, leading to a higher risk of falls. Physical rehabilitation is commonly offered to patients undergoing TJR to optimize postoperative outcomes, including strength, physical function, pain reduction, and return to normal activities of daily living. Increasingly, "prehabilitation" (rehabilitation services provided before surgery) is also considered to maximize patients' functional status before surgery and improve postoperative outcomes.

IMPORTANCE OF PREHABILITATION AND REHABILITATION

The topic of prehabilitation and rehabilitation (hereafter "(p)rehabilitation") is of interest to health systems to enable evidence-based decision-making regarding which interventions should be offered to adults undergoing TJR for OA. This aims to achieve the best clinical outcomes, reduce avoidable complications or joint failures, and be cost- and resource-effective for the health system, patients, and their caregivers. The Agency for Healthcare Research and Quality's (AHRQ) Learning Health System Panel nominated this topic as of particular interest.

REHABILITATION TIMING AND EFFECTIVENESS

Rehabilitation after TJR is the most common practice in the United States for those who have undergone a TKA or THA procedure. Successful rehabilitation improves pain control, walking and gait, balance, and strength and reduces length of stay. Though less commonly used, prehabilitation (before surgery) has also been recommended. Preoperative health status is a strong predictor of favorable postoperative outcomes, including reduced pain and improved functioning. Thus, prehabilitation is hypothesized to halt further joint deterioration in the preoperative period and accelerate the improvement of function and strength postoperatively. However, the effectiveness of prehabilitation in TJR is unclear. A 2017 systematic review on prehabilitation for TKA or THA found conflicting evidence, with some studies finding no added benefit and others finding improvements in postoperative function, quadriceps strength, and length of stay. A subsequent review of prehabilitation for patients about to undergo

TKA found prehabilitation was associated with decreased length of stay. At the same time, limited data suggested prehabilitation made no difference in patient-reported outcomes of pain or function, stiffness, and physical role.

FACTORS AFFECTING REHABILITATION PROGRAMS

Rehabilitation programs are complex interventions that incorporate multiple specific interventions (modalities) and involve various rehabilitation specialists and personnel, orthopedic surgeons, other clinicians, caregivers, and the patient. Rehabilitation services can occur at different times (i.e., before or after surgery) and in different settings. Rehabilitation is commonly personalized for individuals based on their specific circumstances and response to surgery and rehabilitation. These factors are likely important determinants of the effectiveness of rehabilitation programs to improve strength and mobility, reduce pain, and return the patient to their best possible overall function. However, they all have cost and resource use implications related to the features of the rehabilitation program, the personnel involved, and the location of services. Thus, there are four interrelated considerations in deciding on a rehabilitation program:

- **Timing**. Rehabilitation can occur before surgery (prehabilitation) or after.
- **Type**. Rehabilitation may comprise various types or modalities (e.g., strength training, education, balance training) delivered alone or in combination.
- **Setting**. Rehabilitation may occur in various settings (e.g., acute inpatient, supervised nursing facility, home-based).
- **Cost and resource use**. Each aspect of a rehabilitation program has its associated costs (e.g., due to specialized personnel, equipment, facility overhead).

COMPONENTS OF (P)REHABILITATION PROGRAMS

Prehabilitation and rehabilitation are complex interventions with many facets typically individualized for patients' needs, goals, capabilities, and personalities. The type of (p)rehabilitation includes various concepts: what the intervention is, how it is implemented, and who delivers it. The overall intervention program may include various modalities (typically in combination) to improve a range of body function and structure, and activity and participation domains. These domains have been defined by the International Classification of Functioning, Disability and Health (ICF). They include modalities designed to improve the mobility and stability of joint function, movement control, power and tone of muscles, gait, and endurance, along with the related goal of reducing pain. Examples of modalities include stretching exercises to improve joint mobility, using weights to improve muscle tone, power, and endurance, and stair-climbing to improve mobility, muscle power, movement control, and gait.

In addition to the modalities that directly affect the ICF domains, numerous adjunctive modalities help the patient better achieve their rehabilitation goals. Examples include cryotherapy to reduce swelling and acute pain, mindfulness programs to reduce stress, anxiety, and pain, neuromuscular electrical stimulation (NMES), and biofeedback devices to provide positive incentives. Each modality and the intervention as a whole may vary in how it is delivered, for example, the duration of each session (and the use of each modality within a session), the intensity of the intervention (e.g., minimal vs. maximal extension of range of motion, fewer vs. more repetitions), and the overall duration of the program (e.g., 1 week vs. 2 months before surgery). Further complicating the types of (p)rehabilitation, the overall intervention (or the various modality components) may be delivered by different professionals, ancillary trained personnel, or the patients (or their caregivers) themselves.

DEFINING (P)REHABILITATION

Given the wide range of potential activities that may fall within the concept of (p)rehabilitation, it is challenging to determine what counts as a form of (p)rehabilitation. To focus on the primary interests of the nominating health systems, we focus on structured interventions that involve health professionals or other trained individuals. Thus, for the purpose of this review, we define (p)rehabilitation as active, structured physical activities designed to attain measurable goals of improving impairments and movement-related function as defined by the ICF. The intervention must be delivered, supervised, and/or monitored by a health-care professional or other trained individual, and the patient must be actively involved (i.e., not simply a passive recipient). Pharmaceutical and over-the-counter (OTC) interventions are outside the scope of interest.

SETTINGS FOR (P)REHABILITATION

Another important aspect of (p)rehabilitation is the setting in which it may be delivered. These vary widely, and examples include the acute hospital setting (i.e., immediately postoperative), a skilled nursing facility, an outpatient rehabilitation facility, the patient's home, or a local community center or gym. Interventions may also be delivered virtually by internet, teleconference, web app, or device app. Various factors contribute to deciding the setting (p)rehabilitation will be delivered, such as patient needs, caregiver support, and specific modalities employed. The cost of (p)rehabilitation services, largely determined by setting, plays a major role in deciding which services to provide. In the inpatient setting, "accelerated" rehabilitation after TKA has been associated with reduced length of stay from the acute hospital setting. The effect of the setting of diverse types of (p)rehabilitation programs on patient outcomes is unclear, with some research suggesting facility-based rehabilitation does not provide better recovery compared to home programs for uncomplicated TKA and THA patients, and other evidence suggesting early outpatient rehabilitation may lead to more rapid gains in function, strength, and reduced pain in the short term.

Insurance status may influence patient preference for the setting of care, such that patients under public insurance may be more likely to utilize home-based rehabilitation programs (supervised or unsupervised) over more resource-intensive facility-based rehabilitation programs (including inpatient rehabilitation and outpatient-based sessions). Although facility-based programs are more likely to have skilled, supervised personnel deliver services, evidence of the added benefit of a supervised program remains unclear.

COST CONSIDERATIONS

The total direct costs of care for a TJR episode include the preoperative period (for assessment and, if used, prehabilitation), operative (acute), and postoperative (postacute) periods, with as much as 40 percent of the cost occurring after discharge (70 percent of which are from postacute care facilities). Both operative and postoperative costs (for the health systems, payers, and patients) vary greatly throughout the United States without notable differences in outcomes. As much as a six-fold difference has been observed in the cost of care (from the perspective of the health system) for patients discharged to various types of postacute care, despite similarities in patient characteristics, readmission, and complication rates. TJR of the lower extremity (both THA and TKA) was the most prevalent clinical episode participating in the Centers for Medicare & Medicaid Services (CMS) bundled payment model. As major joint replacement surgeries and bundled payment models become more prevalent, many health systems and payers are working to understand how best to implement the most effective and cost-effective care for TJR patients without compromising their outcomes.

CONCLUSION

Optimizing outcomes in total joint replacement through effective prehabilitation and rehabilitation is crucial for improving patient recovery and QOL. Understanding the importance of timing, types, and settings of rehabilitation programs helps tailor individualized care. Despite the complexities and costs associated with these programs, their role in enhancing strength, mobility, and overall function cannot be understated. Future research and implementation of best practices in (p)rehabilitation will be essential for achieving the best clinical and cost-effective outcomes for patients undergoing total joint replacement.[1]

[1] Effective Health Care Program, "Prehabilitation and Rehabilitation for Major Joint Replacement Surgery," Agency for Healthcare Research and Quality (AHRQ), January 2023. Available online. URL: https://effectivehealthcare.ahrq.gov/products/major-joint-replacement/protocol#field_report_title_4. Accessed July 1, 2024.

Chapter 34 | **Post-Surgery Care after Amputation or Other Surgery**

Taking care of yourself after an amputation or other surgeries is crucial to prevent infections. Any wound or cut from amputation or surgery can get infected if germs or dirt enter your body through an opening in your skin. After your surgery, pay attention to your body and watch for the following signs of infection:

- warmth
- redness and swelling
- white or yellow pus coming out of the wound or cut
- red lines under your skin running up towards your chest from the wound or cut
- sudden increase in pain
- soreness or tenderness that hurts a lot

CARE INSTRUCTIONS

Take good care of the part of your limb that is left, especially the cut where the limb was removed. Infection can lead to severe problems, additional surgeries, or even death. If you suspect an infection, address it immediately by following your nurse's or doctor's instructions. If prescribed antibiotics, complete the entire course, even if the redness or soreness improves.

- Try to rest whenever possible.
- Elevate your limb higher than your chest if you can. This will aid in healing.

WHEN TO SEEK MEDICAL HELP

Seek medical help immediately if you notice any of the following:

- cold or cool skin or limb
- wound or area that smells bad
- feeling very tired or achy
- sore or cut has a thick brown or gray discharge
- skin around the sore or cut turns black or appears unhealthy

PREVENTING INFECTIONS

The best way to handle an infection is to prevent it. Here are some preventive measures:

- Wash your limb with mild soap and clean water, then rinse and pat dry. Do this every day or more often if you sweat a lot or if it is red or sore.
- Wash anything that touches your skin, like socks, with mild soap and clean water, then rinse and dry. Avoid putting wet socks or other clothes on your arm or leg.
- Use lotion to avoid flaking, peeling, and dry skin. Apply lotion at night before going to bed. If you do not have any lotion, use fresh vegetable cooking oil, such as coconut or olive oil. Never use lard or cooking oil.
- Eat healthy foods and drink plenty of water to keep your skin healthy.

By following these guidelines and taking proactive steps, you can significantly reduce the risk of infection and promote a healthy recovery after amputation or other surgeries.[1]

[1] "Take Care of Yourself after an Amputation or Other Surgery," Centers for Disease Control and Prevention (CDC), February 18, 2010. Available online. URL: www2c.cdc.gov/podcasts/media/pdf/TakeCareAfterAmpOrSurgery_Pod.pdf. Accessed July 1, 2024.

Chapter 35 | Understanding and Using Ventilators

WHAT IS A VENTILATOR?

A mechanical ventilator, also known as a "breathing machine," helps you breathe or get enough oxygen into your blood if you have respiratory failure. These machines act as bellows to move air in and out of your lungs. Your respiratory therapist and doctor will set the ventilator to control how often it pushes air into your lungs and how much you receive.

You may be fitted with a mask to get air from the ventilator into your lungs. For more serious breathing problems, you may need a breathing tube. When you are ready to be taken off the ventilator, your health-care team will "wean" you by decreasing ventilator support until you can breathe on your own.

Mechanical ventilators are primarily used in hospitals and transport systems such as ambulances and MEDEVAC air transport. In some cases, they can be used at home if the illness is long term and caregivers receive proper training and have adequate nursing and other resources. Being on a ventilator may increase the risk of pneumonia, vocal cord damage, or other complications.

The Figure 35.1 shows a standard setup for a mechanical ventilator in a hospital room. The ventilator pushes warm, moist air (or air with extra oxygen) to the patient through a breathing tube (also called an "endotracheal tube") or a tightly fitting mask.

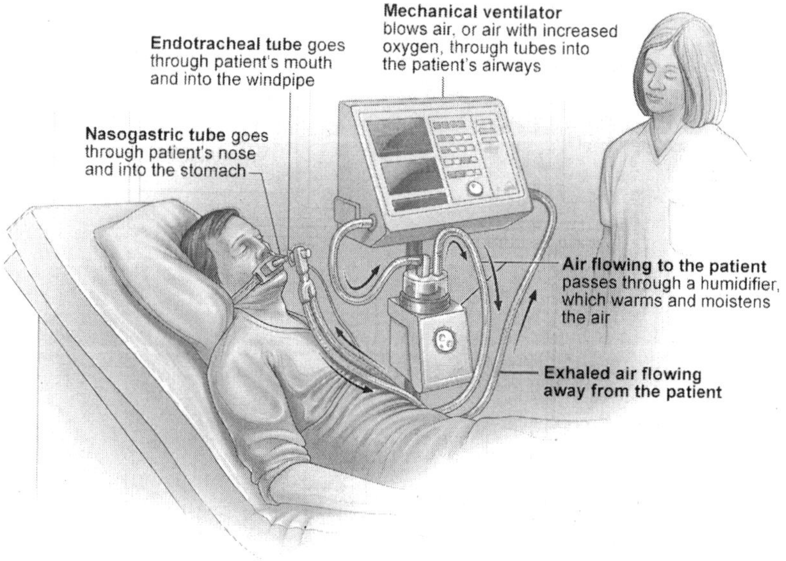

Figure 35.1. Mechanical Ventilator

National Heart, Lung, and Blood Institute (NHLBI)

WHO NEEDS A VENTILATOR?

Respiratory Failure

Respiratory failure is a life-threatening emergency where your organs do not get enough oxygen to function properly. Conditions that may lead to respiratory failure include:

- acute respiratory distress syndrome (ARDS)
- head injury or stroke
- asthma
- chronic obstructive pulmonary disease (COPD) or other lung diseases
- cardiac arrest
- drug overdose
- neonatal respiratory distress syndrome
- pneumonia

- sepsis (infection in the bloodstream)
- spinal cord injuries, polio, amyotrophic lateral sclerosis (ALS), myasthenia gravis, and other diseases affecting nerves and muscles involved in breathing

Surgery

You may need a ventilator during surgery with general anesthesia, as the medicines used can affect your normal breathing. A ventilator helps control your breathing during the procedure.

WHAT TO EXPECT

Ventilators blow air into your airways and lungs, carrying oxygen-rich air in and carbon dioxide out. They can be set to "breathe" a set number of times per minute or assist only when you need help breathing.

Before being put on a ventilator, you may receive:

- oxygen through a mask
- medicines to make you sleepy and stop you from feeling pain
- fluids and other medicines through an IV to help keep oxygen-rich blood flowing to your organs

There are two ways to get air from the ventilator into your lungs: through a face mask or a breathing tube.

Ventilation with a Face Mask

Noninvasive ventilation with a face mask fits tightly over your nose and mouth to help you breathe. This method is recommended if your breathing problems are not severe enough for a breathing tube or to help you transition to breathing on your own after a breathing tube is removed.

Benefits of face mask ventilation include:

- greater comfort compared to a breathing tube
- ability to cough
- ability to talk and swallow

- reduced need for sedative and pain medicines
- lower risk of pneumonia associated with breathing tubes

Ventilation with a Breathing Tube

For more serious cases, you may need invasive ventilation with a breathing tube placed into your windpipe, connected to a ventilator that blows air directly into your airways. The process of inserting the tube is called "intubation." The tube is typically inserted through your nose or mouth and moved down into your throat and windpipe. It is held in place by tape or a strap around your head.

In some cases, especially for long-term ventilation, a tracheostomy may be performed. In this procedure, a hole is made in the neck to insert a tube directly into the windpipe. This tube, called a "trach" tube, is more comfortable for longer use and allows some speech and eating.

WHAT TO EXPECT WHILE ON A VENTILATOR

Being on a ventilator is not usually painful but can be uncomfortable. With a breathing tube, you will not be able to eat or talk. With a trach tube, you may be able to talk with a special device and eat some types of food. With a face mask, you will be able to talk and eat if recommended by your health-care team.

Ventilators limit movement and may keep you in bed. Your health-care team will closely monitor you, with regular lung imaging tests and blood tests to check oxygen and carbon dioxide levels. Adjustments to the ventilator's airflow and settings will be made as needed.

ONGOING CARE

A respiratory therapist or nurse will suction your breathing tube to remove mucus from your lungs, causing brief shortness of breath and coughing. You may receive nutrients through an IV or a feeding tube. For long-term ventilation, a tracheostomy may be done, and you may be given a portable ventilator to allow movement and outdoor activities.

WHAT TO EXPECT WHEN TAKEN OFF A VENTILATOR

After surgery, your health-care team will disconnect the ventilator once you start breathing on your own. Weaning involves gradually decreasing ventilator support. Most people can breathe on their own after the first weaning attempt. If you cannot, repeated weaning attempts will be made. If long-term ventilation is required, you may need a tracheostomy and a portable ventilator.

RISKS OF BEING ON A VENTILATOR

Being on a ventilator can increase the risk of:

- infections, such as pneumonia and sinus infections
- atelectasis (collapsed air sacs)
- blood clots and bedsores
- pulmonary edema (fluid in the air sacs)
- lung damage from excessive air or pressure
- pneumothorax (air leakage into the chest)
- vocal cord damage
- weakened diaphragm and breathing muscles

GOING HOME ON A VENTILATOR

If long-term ventilation is needed, you may use a ventilator at home, improving quality of life (QOL) and avoiding some hospital complications. Your health-care team will train you and your caregivers on using and maintaining the ventilator, recognizing serious problems, and when to call for help. You may need additional equipment, such as a back-up ventilator, oxygen tank, suction machine, humidifier, pulse oximeter, and nebulizer.

USING YOUR VENTILATOR AT HOME

Regular equipment checks and good hygiene practices are essential. Keep records of symptoms and respond quickly to ventilator alarms. Avoid secondhand smoke and get routine vaccinations.

FOLLOW-UP CARE

Your health-care team will provide follow-up care, including home visits and adjustments to your treatment. Notify utility companies if someone in your household is on a ventilator to ensure quick service restoration during outages. Keep a list of health conditions, treatments, and medicines for emergencies.[1]

[1] "What Is a Ventilator?" National Heart, Lung, and Blood Institute (NHLBI), March 24, 2022. Available online. URL: www.nhlbi.nih.gov/health/ventilator. Accessed July 18, 2024.

Chapter 36 | Ostomy Care after Surgery

Living with an ostomy can be overwhelming and scary for some people. However, most people adjust and lead active and productive lives. A wound, ostomy, and continence (WOC) nurse or an enterostomal therapist will provide education, support, and medical advice on topics that include the following:

- what to expect after ostomy surgery
- caring for an ostomy
- resuming normal activities after ostomy surgery
- maintaining personal relationships after ostomy surgery
- coping with practical, social, and emotional issues

WHAT TO EXPECT AFTER OSTOMY SURGERY

Once the person is home from the hospital, the first week or two are considered an extension of the hospital stay. Most people will tire quite easily when they first come home. Getting enough rest is important. Gradually, stamina and strength will improve. Most people can return to work about six to eight weeks after surgery. People may have certain gastrointestinal (GI) issues—such as gas, diarrhea, and constipation—as the bowel heals, depending on the type of bowel diversion.

Ileostomy and Colostomy

People with an ileostomy or a colostomy may have excessive gas during the early weeks and months after surgery. This extra gas will decrease once the bowel has had time to heal and the person resumes a regular diet.

Ileoanal Reservoir

People with an ileoanal reservoir initially have about 6–10 bowel movements a day. The newly formed ileoanal reservoir takes several months to stretch and adjust to its new function. After the adjustment period, bowel movements decrease to as few as four to six a day. People with an ileoanal reservoir may have mild fecal incontinence and may have to get up during periods of sleep to pass stool.

Continent Ileostomy

Similar to people with an ileostomy or a colostomy, people with a continent ileostomy may have excessive gas during the early weeks and months after surgery.

CARING FOR AN OSTOMY

During the recovery in the hospital and at home, a person will learn to care for the ostomy. The type of care required depends on the type of ostomy surgery. A WOC nurse or an enterostomal therapist will teach a person about special care after ostomy surgery.

Ileostomy and Colostomy

People with an ileostomy or a colostomy will learn how to attach, drain, and change their ostomy pouch and care for the stoma and the surrounding skin. Ostomy pouches, or pouching systems, may be one piece or two pieces. They include a barrier, also called a "wafer" or "flange," and a disposable plastic pouch. In a two-piece system, the pouch can be detached or replaced without removing the barrier. For both systems, the barrier attaches to the skin around the stoma and protects it from stool. The length of time the barrier stays sealed to the skin depends on many things, such as:

- how well the barrier fits
- the condition of the skin around the stoma
- the person's level of physical activity
- the shape of the body around the stoma

Most people can leave the barrier on for three to seven days. However, a person should change the barrier as soon as stool starts to go underneath it and onto the skin.

Most ostomy pouches empty through an opening in the bottom. Emptying the pouch several times a day reduces the chance of leakage and bulges underneath the person's clothing. A person should empty the pouch when it is about one-third full. He or she should rinse the pouch in a two-piece system before reattaching it to the skin barrier.

How often a person needs to change his or her pouching system depends on the type of system. Many pouching systems may be worn for three to seven days. Some pouching systems are made to be changed every day. When changing a pouch system, the person should:

- wipe away any mucus on the stoma
- clean the skin around the stoma with warm water and a washcloth
- rinse the skin thoroughly
- dry the skin completely

People may use mild soap to clean the skin. However, the soap should not have oils, perfumes, or deodorants, which may cause skin problems or keep the skin barrier from sticking. A WOC nurse or an enterostomal therapist can give advice if a person has problems attaching the skin barrier or keeping it attached.

When changing the pouching system, people should inspect the stoma and contact a health-care provider about any dramatic changes in stoma size, shape, or color. People should look for blood and signs of skin irritation around the stoma. Sensitivities or allergies to ostomy products such as adhesives, skin barriers, pastes, tape, or pouch materials can cause skin irritation. People with pouching systems can test different products to see if their skin reacts to them. People should use only ostomy products recommended by their health-care provider.

Ileoanal Reservoir

People with an ileoanal reservoir will learn how to care for irritated skin around the anus resulting from frequent stools or fecal incontinence. A WOC nurse or an enterostomal therapist may recommend pelvic floor exercises to help strengthen the muscles around the anus.

Continent Ileostomy

People with a continent ileostomy will learn how to insert a catheter through the stoma to drain the internal pouch. They can drain the pouch by standing in front of the toilet or by sitting on the restroom and then emptying the catheter. During the first few weeks after a continent ileostomy, the person needs to drain the internal pouch about every two hours. After a few weeks, the person is able to go four to six hours between pouch drainings. The person should wash his or her hands with soap and water after using a catheter. The person should clean the skin around the stoma with warm water and a washcloth and let the skin dry completely.

Living with an ostomy can be challenging, but with proper education and support from health-care professionals, individuals can lead active and fulfilling lives. Adapting to the changes and following the recommended care routines will help manage the ostomy effectively and maintain a good quality of life (QOL).[1]

[1] "Ostomy Surgery of the Bowel," National Institute of Diabetes and Digestive and Kidney Diseases (NIDDK), July 2014. Available online. URL: www.niddk.nih.gov/-/media/Files/Digestive-Diseases/Ostomy_Surgery_508.pdf. Accessed April 9, 2024.

Chapter 37 | Recovery and Rehabilitation after Heart Surgery

Heart surgery is done to correct problems with the heart. Your provider may recommend surgery after lifestyle changes, medicines, or other procedures no longer work. Heart surgery may also be done in an emergency situation, such as a heart attack. Each year, more than 2 million people around the world have open-heart surgery to treat various heart problems.

RECOVERY IN THE HOSPITAL

After your surgery, you may spend a day or more in the hospital's intensive care unit (ICU), depending on the type of surgery you had. An intravenous (IV) needle might be inserted in a blood vessel in your arm or chest to give you fluids until you're ready to drink on your own. Your health-care team may also give you extra oxygen through a face mask or nasal prongs that fit just inside your nose. They will remove the mask or prongs when you no longer need them.

When you leave the ICU, you will be moved to another part of the hospital for several days before you go home. While in the hospital, your health-care team will closely monitor your heart rate, blood pressure, breathing, and incision sites.

RECOVERY AT HOME

People respond differently to heart surgery. Your recovery at home will depend on the type of heart problem and surgery you had, as well as your overall health. Before you go home, your provider will tell you how to:

- care for your healing incision(s)
- recognize signs of infection or other complications
- cope with the after-effects of surgery

Your health-care team will give you information about follow-up appointments, medicines, and situations when you should call your provider right away. They will also let you know when to expect to resume daily activities such as driving and working.

Discomfort and some pain after heart surgery are normal. Your provider will work with you to provide medicine to ease any pain you may feel. Some common after-effects of heart surgery include:

- constipation, especially if you are taking pain medicine
- difficulty sleeping
- loss of appetite
- memory problems
- mood swings or depression
- pain in your chest or muscles, especially if you have an incision in your leg from coronary artery bypass grafting (CABG)

ONGOING CARE AND RECOVERY

You will need to see your provider regularly to monitor your recovery and take steps to prevent another heart problem.

- **Schedule regular checkups**. Checkups with your provider or surgeon are an essential part of your ongoing care after heart surgery. During these visits, you may have blood tests or heart tests such as an electrocardiogram (ECG or EKG), echocardiography, or a stress test. These tests will show how your heart is working after the surgery.
- **Take your medicine as prescribed**. Depending on your condition and type of heart procedure, you may need to take a blood-thinning medicine for several months following your surgery.

- **Make heart-healthy lifestyle changes.** Your provider may recommend lifestyle changes to help you stay healthy. For example, your provider may advise you to quit smoking, choose heart-healthy foods, be physically active (when it is safe), manage stress, and get enough good quality sleep.
- **Learn more about how to protect your heart and prevent future problems.** Depending on the type of heart surgery, your provider may refer you to cardiac rehabilitation. Cardiac rehabilitation is a medically supervised program for people recovering from heart problems. It usually includes exercise training, education on heart-healthy living, and counseling to reduce stress and help you recover. Your provider can help you find a cardiac rehabilitation program near your home.[1]

CARDIAC REHABILITATION

Cardiac rehabilitation is a supervised program that includes physical activity, health education, and counseling to help individuals recovering from a heart attack, heart failure, or other cardiac event that required surgery or medical care. It includes:

- exercise counseling and training
- lifestyle education
- counseling to reduce stress

Cardiac rehabilitation can benefit men and women, people of all ages, and people with varying levels of heart problems. It can strengthen the heart and body after a heart attack, relieve post-cardiac event symptoms, relieve stress, improve mental health, and build healthier habits, such as increased physical activity, quitting smoking, and following a heart-healthy diet.

Cardiac rehabilitation can be delivered by a team of professionals, including patients' health-care teams, exercise and nutrition specialists, physical therapists, and counselors.

---

[1] "Heart Surgery: Recovery," National Heart, Lung, and Blood Institute (NHLBI), June 1, 2022. Available online. URL: www.nhlbi.nih.gov/health/heart-surgery/recovery. Accessed July 19, 2024.

Cardiac rehabilitation plays a crucial role in the recovery process, offering structured support and resources to help you build and maintain healthier habits for a better quality of life (QOL).[2]

[2] "Cardiac Rehabilitation to Support Recovery from Cardiac Events," Centers for Disease Control and Prevention (CDC), May 24, 2024. Available online. URL: https://hdsbpc.cdc.gov/s/article/Cardiac-Rehabilitation-to-Support-Recovery-from-Cardiac-Events. Accessed July 19, 2024.

Chapter 38 | **Reducing the Risk of Blood Clots during Long-Distance Travel**

OVERVIEW

More than 300 million people travel on long-distance flights (generally more than four hours) each year. Blood clots, also called "deep vein thrombosis" (DVT), can be a serious risk for some long-distance travelers. Most information about blood clots and long-distance travel comes from air travel data. However, anyone traveling more than four hours, whether by air, car, bus, or train, can be at risk for blood clots.

Blood clots can form in the deep veins of your legs during travel because you are sitting still in a confined space for long periods. The longer you are immobile, the greater your risk of developing a blood clot. A DVT occurs when a blood clot forms in the deep veins of the legs. Sometimes, the blood clot dissolves on its own. However, a serious health problem can occur when a part of the blood clot breaks off and travels to the lungs, causing a blockage called a "pulmonary embolism" (PE), which can be fatal. The good news is that there are steps you can take to protect your health and reduce your risk of blood clots during a long-distance trip.

RISK FACTORS FOR BLOOD CLOTS

Even if you travel a long distance, the risk of developing a blood clot is generally very small. Your risk level depends on the duration of travel and whether you have any other risks for blood clots. Most people who develop travel-associated blood clots have one or more other risk factors, such as:

- older age (risk increases after age 40)
- overweight or obesity
- recent surgery or injury (within three months)
- use of estrogen-containing contraceptives (e.g., birth control pills, rings, patches)
- hormone replacement therapy (treatment to reduce menopause effects)
- pregnancy and the postpartum period (up to three months after childbirth)
- a previous blood clot
- inherited blood clotting disorder
- family history of blood clots
- active cancer or recent cancer treatment
- certain other long-term conditions (e.g., heart or lung conditions, diabetes)
- limited mobility (e.g., a leg cast)
- catheter placed in a large vein
- varicose veins

The combination of long-distance travel with one or more of these risks may increase the likelihood of developing a blood clot. The more risks you have, the greater your chances of experiencing a blood clot. If you plan on traveling soon, talk with your doctor to learn more about what you can do to protect your health. The most important thing you can do is to learn and recognize the symptoms of blood clots.

RECOGNIZING THE SYMPTOMS

Deep Vein Thrombosis

About half of people with DVT have no symptoms at all. The following are the most common symptoms of DVT that occur in the affected part of the body (usually the leg or arm):

- swelling of your leg or arm
- pain or tenderness that you can't explain

- skin that is warm to the touch
- redness or discoloration of the skin

If you have any of these symptoms, contact your doctor immediately.

Pulmonary Embolism

You can have a PE without any symptoms of a DVT. Symptoms of a PE can include:

- difficulty breathing
- faster than normal or irregular heartbeat
- chest pain or discomfort, which usually worsens with a deep breath or coughing
- anxiety
- cough or coughing up blood
- lightheadedness or fainting

If you have any of these symptoms, seek medical help immediately.

PROTECTING YOURSELF DURING TRAVEL

- **Know what to look for**. Be alert to the signs and symptoms of blood clots.
- **Talk with your doctor**. If you think you may be at risk for blood clots, discuss it with your doctor. If you have had a previous blood clot or if a family member has a history of blood clots or an inherited clotting disorder, learn more about your individual risks.
- **Move your legs frequently**. On long trips, exercise your calf muscles to improve blood flow. If you've been sitting for a long time, take a break to stretch your legs. Extend your legs straight out and flex your ankles (pulling your toes toward you). Some airlines suggest pulling each knee toward the chest, holding it there with your hands on your lower leg for 15 seconds, and repeating up to 10 times. These activities help to improve blood flow in your legs.

- **Consider compression stockings.** If you are at risk, talk with your doctor about wearing graduated compression stockings.
- **Follow medication guidelines.** If you are on blood thinners (anticoagulants), follow your doctor's recommendations on medication use.

By taking these precautions, you can reduce your risk of developing blood clots during long-distance travel and ensure a safer journey.[1]

[1] "Understanding Your Risk for Blood Clots with Travel," Centers for Disease Control and Prevention (CDC), May 15, 2024. Available online. URL: www.cdc.gov/blood-clots/risk-factors/travel.html. Accessed July 19, 2024.

Chapter 39 | Effective Hospital Discharge Planning

Hospital discharge planning is a critical component in the transition from hospital to home. Effective discharge planning helps reduce the likelihood of readmissions and ensures that patients receive the necessary follow-up care. This chapter provides an overview of the IDEAL Discharge Planning strategy, which focuses on engaging patients and their families in the discharge process.

THE IDEAL DISCHARGE PLANNING STRATEGY

The IDEAL Discharge Planning strategy is designed to actively involve patients and their families in the discharge process. The goal is to ensure a safe and effective transition from hospital to home. The strategy includes the following key elements:

- Include the patient and family as full partners in the discharge planning process:
  - Involve them in team meetings about discharge.
  - Identify which family members or friends will provide care at home.
- Discuss with the patient and family five key areas to prevent problems at home:
  - Describe what life at home will be like, including the home environment, support needed, dietary restrictions, and activities to avoid.
  - Review medications, including their purpose, dosage, administration, and potential side effects.

    - Highlight warning signs and problems, providing contact information for someone to call if issues arise.
    - Explain test results and what they mean for the patient's health.
    - Make follow-up appointments and ensure the patient and family know the details.
- Educate the patient and family in plain language about the patient's condition, the discharge process, and next steps:
    - Provide information throughout the hospital stay, not just at discharge.
    - Use teach-back methods to ensure understanding.
- Assess how well doctors and nurses explain the diagnosis, condition, and next steps:
    - Use small chunks of information and repeat key points.
    - Ask the patient and family to repeat back what they understood.
- Listen to and honor the patient and family's goals, preferences, observations, and concerns:
    - Encourage the use of a whiteboard in the room for questions or concerns.
    - Schedule at least one meeting specific to discharge planning.

TOOLS FOR IDEAL DISCHARGE PLANNING

Several tools are available to support the IDEAL Discharge Planning strategy:

IDEAL Discharge Planning Overview, Process, and Checklist

- used by clinicians to keep track of the discharge process
- includes an overview, process steps, and a checklist for each patient

Be Prepared to Go Home Checklist and Booklet

- given to patients soon after admission
- helps identify and discuss questions and concerns about going home

Improving Discharge Outcomes with Patients and Families

- informs physicians of the IDEAL Discharge Planning process
- distributed at staff meetings or other venues

Care Transitions from Hospital to Home: IDEAL Discharge Planning Training

- prepares clinicians and hospital staff to engage patients and families in discharge planning
- includes a PowerPoint presentation and talking points

IMPLEMENTING IDEAL DISCHARGE PLANNING

Implementing the IDEAL Discharge Planning strategy involves several steps:

- Form a multidisciplinary team.
  - Include hospital leaders, physicians, nurses, other clinical and management staff, and patient and family representatives.
- Assess current views on the discharge process.
  - Review current discharge planning steps, strengths, and areas for improvement.
  - Engage patients and families in identifying challenges and solutions.
- Set aims to improve discharge planning.
  - Define specific, measurable goals.
  - Examples include implementing IDEAL tools in multiple units or reducing readmissions by a certain percentage.
- Decide on how to implement the strategy.
  - Adapt the IDEAL Discharge Planning process and tools to fit the hospital environment.
  - Clarify roles and responsibilities for each team member.
- Train staff.
  - Conduct training sessions for all staff involved in the discharge process.

  - Use a mix of teaching methods, including role play and feedback.
- Distribute tools and incorporate key principles into practice.
  - Ensure all clinicians and hospital staff include patients and families in the discharge planning process.
  - Provide ongoing support and feedback.
- Evaluate implementation.
  - Monitor the discharge process and provide feedback to staff.
  - Gather feedback from patients, families, and staff to refine the process.

CASE STUDY: ADVOCATE TRINITY HOSPITAL

Advocate Trinity Hospital implemented IDEAL Discharge Planning as part of a pilot project. Key elements of their success included:

- **Staff ownership**. Engaging unit-based councils and assigning implementation roles to staff.
- **Training**. Using a train-the-trainer model to prepare staff.
- **Monitoring and support**. Conducting weekly huddles to discuss challenges and ensure effective discharge planning.

As a result, Advocate Trinity Hospital saw improved patient satisfaction scores and better discharge outcomes. The IDEAL Discharge Planning strategy helped nurses become more aware of patients' needs and improved communication with patients and families.

CONCLUSION

Effective hospital discharge planning is essential for ensuring patients' safety and reducing readmissions. The IDEAL Discharge Planning strategy provides a comprehensive approach to engaging patients and families in the discharge process. By involving patients and families as full partners and using clear communication, hospitals can improve the transition from hospital to home and enhance patient outcomes.[1]

[1] "Care Transitions from Hospital to Home: IDEAL Discharge Planning Implementation Handbook," Agency for Healthcare Research and Quality (AHRQ), December 4, 2017. Available online. URL: www.ahrq.gov/sites/default/files/wysiwyg/professionals/systems/hospital/engagingfamilies/strategy4/Strat4_Implement_Hndbook_508_v2.pdf. Accessed July 19, 2024.

Chapter 40 | Choosing and Transitioning to Nursing Home Care

OVERVIEW OF NURSING HOME CARE

Nursing home care can be divided into custodial care, such as assistance with bathing or dressing, and skilled care, such as changing sterile bandages. People go to nursing homes for various reasons, including illness, injury recovery, post-surgery rehabilitation, or chronic care needs requiring ongoing nursing care.

Long-term care encompasses medical and nonmedical assistance for those unable to perform basic activities of daily living (ADLs), such as dressing or bathing. Long-term support can be provided at home, in the community, in assisted living facilities, or in nursing homes.

Before choosing a nursing home, explore other options available, including community services, home care, or assisted living, depending on your needs and resources.

UNDERSTANDING MEDICARE AND MEDICAID COVERAGE

If You Have Medicare

Medicare Part A (Hospital Insurance) may cover:

- care in a certified skilled nursing facility (SNF) if medically necessary for skilled care
- short-term nursing stays following hospitalization
- limited home- and community-based long-term care

Part A does not cover:

- custodial care if it is the only care needed
- long-term care or stays in a nursing home

If You Have Medicaid

Medicaid may cover long-term nursing home stays and home—and community-based services. These services allow people with Medicaid to receive care in their homes or community-based settings. Medicaid programs serve various groups, including those with mental illnesses, intellectual or developmental disabilities, and/or physical disabilities.

CHOOSING A NURSING HOME

Step 1: Find Nursing Homes in Your Area

- Ask people you trust, such as family, friends, or neighbors.
- Ask your doctor if they provide care at any local nursing homes.
- Visit www.medicare.gov/care-compare/?providerType=NursingHome.
- Use the Eldercare Locator or an Aging and Disability Resource Center (ADRC).
- Contact your local senior and community activity center.
- If in the hospital, ask your social worker about discharge planning as early as possible.

Step 2: Compare the Quality of the Nursing Homes You Are Considering

- Visit Nursing Home Compare to get information on the quality of Medicare- and Medicaid-certified nursing homes.
- Consider the information carefully, along with other information you gather, to guide your decision.

Resources for choosing a nursing home:

- Call your Long-Term Care (LTC) Ombudsman.
- Call your state health department or state licensing agency for written information on the quality of care in local nursing homes.

- Please look at the survey findings (CMS Form 2567) for the facility on Nursing Home Compare and in the nursing home.

Step 3: Visit the Nursing Homes You Are Interested In

- Visit nursing homes before making a final decision.
- If you cannot visit, ask a family member or friend to visit for you.
- Call and make an appointment to meet with staff, and visit at other times without an appointment.
- Ask questions and talk with residents and their families.
- Write down any questions you have after your visit.

Consider the following during your visit:

- participation in social, recreational, religious, or cultural activities
- provided transportation to community activities
- private spaces for visitors
- continuity of care with personal doctors
- quality of care and staffing information
- CNA-to-resident ratio during each shift
- available therapy types and staff
- types of meals served and dietary accommodations
- access to preventive care and specialists
- screening program for vaccinations
- access to oral and mental health care
- care for people with dementia and policy on antipsychotic medication use

Use the "Nursing Home Checklist" from www.medicare.gov to help evaluate nursing homes.

Step 4: Choose the Nursing Home That Meets Your Needs

- Discuss your options with family, friends, doctor, clergy, or social worker.
- Compare nursing homes if more than one meets your needs.

- If you do not like a nursing home, look at other options.
- If in the hospital and do not like the available nursing home, talk to the discharge planner or doctor for other arrangements.

NEXT STEPS AFTER CHOOSING A NURSING HOME

Information for the Nursing Home Office Staff

- Provide health coverage and long-term care insurance information.
- Understand Medicare and Medicaid rules regarding deposits and charges.

Information for the Nursing Home Medical Staff

- Provide your medical history, current health status, medications, health-care providers, and emergency contacts.

Other Important Information

- Provide health-care advance directives, such as a living will or durable power of attorney for health care.

ONCE YOU ARE A RESIDENT

Information the Nursing Home Must Provide

- Medicare and Medicaid benefits and refunds for covered payments.

Personal Needs Accounts

- Managed by the nursing home for personal use expenses.

Your Assessment and Care Plan

- Nursing home staff will assess your health condition and develop a care plan within 14 days of admission.
- The care plan will include personal and health-care services, equipment, dietary needs, and goals.

Your Resident Rights and Protections

- Residents have rights under federal and state law, including being free from discrimination, abuse, and neglect, and receiving proper medical care.
- The nursing home must communicate these rights in a language and format you understand.

REPORTING AND RESOLVING PROBLEMS

- Talk to the staff involved or follow the facility's grievance procedure.
- Contact the LTC Ombudsman, State Survey Agency, or P&A Agency if needed.
- Visit www.medicare.gov/talk-to-someone or call 800-MEDICARE for contact information.

MOVING TO ANOTHER FACILITY

- If you are unsatisfied with your current nursing home, you can move to another facility with an available bed.
- Discuss the rules for leaving with the nursing home staff.

For more information and resources, visit www.medicare.gov.[1]

[1] "Your Guide to Choosing a Nursing Home or Other Long-Term Services & Supports," Centers for Medicare & Medicaid Services (CMS), October 2019. Available online. URL: www.medicare.gov/care-compare/en/assets/resources/nursing-home/02174-nursing-home-other-long-term-services.pdf. Accessed April 9, 2024.

Part 6 | Additional Help and Information

Chapter 41 | Glossary of Terms Related to Surgery

amputation: Removal of part or all of a body part, except for internal organs. It usually takes place during surgery in a hospital operating room.

aneurysm: A thin or weak spot in an artery that balloons out and can burst.

antibiotic: Drugs used to fight bacteria in the body.

atherosclerosis: A disease in which fatty material is deposited on the wall of the arteries, causing them to narrow and eventually restricting blood flow.

bacteria: Microorganisms that can cause infections.

benign: A tumor or cells that are not cancerous.

biopsy: The removal of body tissues for examination under a microscope or for other tests.

bladder: The organ in the human body that stores urine, located in the lower part of the abdomen.

blood transfusion: A procedure in which a person is given an infusion of whole blood or blood components. The blood may be donated by another person or may have been taken from the patient earlier and stored until needed.

body mass index (BMI): A measure of body weight relative to height. The BMI tool uses a formula that produces a score often used to determine if a person is underweight, at a normal weight, overweight, or obese.

cataracts: Cloudy or thick areas in the lens of the eye.

cholesterol: A fat-like substance made by the body and found naturally in animal foods such as dairy products, eggs, meat, poultry, and seafood.

chronic illness: An illness that persists over a long period of time.

colonoscopy: A procedure that allows a doctor to look inside the large intestine using an instrument with a tiny camera called a "scope."

This glossary contains terms excerpted from documents produced by several sources deemed reliable.

Crohn's disease: An ongoing condition that causes inflammation of the digestive tract, also called the "gastrointestinal (GI) tract." It can affect any part of the GI tract from the mouth to the anus.

elective surgery: A surgery that is optional and not required.

endoscope: A thin, illuminated, flexible, or rigid tube-like optical system used to examine the interior of a hollow organ or body cavity by direct insertion. Instruments can be attached for biopsy and surgery.

estrogen: A hormone made by the body that helps develop and maintain female sex characteristics and the growth of long bones.

exercise: A type of physical activity that is planned and structured, done on purpose to improve or maintain health, physical fitness, and/or physical performance.

fat: A major source of energy in the diet.

fatigue: A feeling of lack of energy, weariness, or tiredness.

gallbladder: A sac that stores bile, a fluid produced by the liver. After eating, bile is secreted into the small intestine to help digest fats.

gastrointestinal: Referring to the stomach and the intestines or bowels.

general surgery: The branch of surgery that covers the main areas of surgical treatment. General surgeons treat diseases of the abdomen, breast, head and neck, blood vessels, and digestive tract. They also manage the care of patients who have been injured or have deformities or other conditions requiring surgery.

glucose: A major source of energy for the body and a building block for many carbohydrates. The digestive process breaks down carbohydrates in foods and drinks into glucose.

heart attack: Also called an "acute myocardial infarction" (AMI). It occurs when one of the heart's arteries becomes blocked, slowing or stopping the supply of blood and oxygen to part of the heart muscle. When the heart muscle does not get the oxygen and nutrients it needs, the affected heart tissue may die.

hormone: A substance produced by one tissue and conveyed by the bloodstream to another to effect a function of the body, such as growth or metabolism.

hypnosis: A focused state of concentration used to reduce pain. With self-hypnosis, a positive statement is repeated over and over. With guided imagery, relaxing images are created in the mind.

hysterectomy: Surgery to remove the uterus and, sometimes, the cervix. When both the uterus and the cervix are removed, it is called a "total hysterectomy." When only the uterus is removed, it is called a "partial hysterectomy."

immune system: The body's natural defense system against infection and disease. White blood cells are the main part of the immune system that fights infections.

incision: A cut made in the body to perform surgery.

infection: A condition when germs enter a person's body and multiply, causing disease. The germs may be bacteria, viruses, yeast, or fungi. When the body's natural defense system is strong, it can often fight the germs and prevent infection. Some cancer treatments can weaken the natural defense system.

kidney stones: Hard masses that develop from crystals separating from the urine and building up on the inner surfaces of the kidney.

larynx: The valve structure between the trachea (windpipe) and the pharynx (upper throat), which is the primary organ of voice production.

long-term care: Services that help meet the medical and nonmedical needs of people with a chronic illness or disability.

malignant: A tumor or cell that is cancerous.

medical error: An unintended but preventable adverse effect of care, whether or not it is evident or harmful to the patient.

medical record: Documentation of a patient's medical history and care.

mortality: Refers to the death rate or the number of deaths in a certain group of people in a certain period.

nonsteroidal anti-inflammatory drugs (NSAIDs): Pain relievers such as aspirin, ibuprofen, and naproxen. These medicines are safe and effective when taken as directed but can cause stomach bleeding or kidney problems in some people.

nutrition: The clinical practice concerned with nutrients and other substances in food and their action, interaction, and balance in relation to health and disease.

pharmacist: A person licensed to prepare and dispense prescription drugs and medicines and who has been trained in how they work, how to use them, and their side effects.

prescription: A direction written by the physician to the pharmacist for the preparation and use of a medicine or remedy.

radiation: The emission of energy as electromagnetic waves or moving subatomic particles, especially high-energy particles that cause ionization.

radiologist: Doctors who specialize in diagnosing and treating diseases and injuries using medical imaging techniques such as x-rays, computed tomography (CT), magnetic resonance imaging (MRI), nuclear medicine, positron emission tomography (PET), and ultrasound.

rehabilitation: In medicine, a process to restore mental and/or physical abilities lost to injury or disease to function in a normal or near-normal way.

side effect: An effect of a drug, chemical, or other medicine that is in addition to its intended effect, especially an effect that is harmful or unpleasant.

spinal block: A small dose of medicine given as a shot into the spinal fluid in the lower back.

surgical site infection: An infection that occurs after surgery in the part of the body where the surgery took place. These infections can sometimes be superficial, involving only the skin. Other surgical site infections are more serious and can involve tissues under the skin, organs, or implanted material.

tracheostomy: A surgical opening into the trachea (windpipe) to help someone breathe who has an obstruction or swelling in the larynx (voice box) or upper throat or who has had the larynx surgically removed.

tumor: An abnormal growth of body tissue. Tumors can be cancerous (malignant) or noncancerous (benign). Cancerous tumors can grow uncontrollably and may spread to other parts of the body. Noncancerous tumors do not grow or spread.

ventilator: In medicine, a machine used to help a patient breathe, also called a "respirator."

viruses: Small microscopic organisms that often cause disease.

x-ray: A type of high-energy radiation. In low doses, x-rays are used to diagnose diseases by making pictures of the inside of the body.

Chapter 42 | Directory of Organizations Providing Information about Surgery

GOVERNMENT ORGANIZATIONS

Agency for Healthcare Research and Quality (AHRQ)
5600 Fishers Ln.
Seventh Fl.
Rockville, MD 20857
Phone: 301-427-1364
Website: www.ahrq.gov

Centers for Disease Control and Prevention (CDC)
1600 Clifton Rd., N.E.
Atlanta, GA 30333
Toll-Free: 800-CDC-INFO
(800-232-4636)
Phone: 404-639-3311
Toll-Free TTY: 888-232-6348
Website: www.cdc.gov

Centers for Medicare & Medicaid Services (CMS)
7500 Security Blvd.
Baltimore, MD 21244
Toll-Free: 800-MEDICARE
(800-633-4227)
Phone: 410-786-3000
Toll-Free TTY: 877-486-2048
Website: www.cms.gov

Federal Trade Commission (FTC)
600 Pennsylvania Ave., N.W.
Washington, DC 20580
Toll-Free: 877-FTC-HELP
(877-382-4357)
Phone: 202-326-2222
Website: www.ftc.gov

Resources here were compiled from several sources deemed reliable; all contact information was verified and updated in August 2024.

Healthfinder®
200 Independence Ave., S.W.
Washington, DC 20201
Website: healthfinder.gov
Email: healthfinder@hhs.gov

National Cancer Institute (NCI)
9609 Medical Center Dr.
Bethesda, MD 20892-9760
Toll-Free: 800-4-CANCER
(800-422-6237)
Website: www.cancer.gov
Email: NCIinfo@nih.gov

National Center for Health Statistics (NCHS)
3311 Toledo Rd.
Hyattsville, MD 20782-2064
Phone: 301-458-4000
Website: www.cdc.gov/nchs

National Eye Institute (NEI)
31 Center Dr., MSC 2510
Bethesda, MD 20892-2510
Phone: 301-496-5248
Website: www.nei.nih.gov
Email: 2020@nei.nih.gov

National Heart, Lung, and Blood Institute (NHLBI)
P.O. Box 30105
Bethesda, MD 20824-0105
Phone: 301-592-8573
TTY: 240-629-3255
Website: www.nhlbi.nih.gov
Email: nhlbiinfo@nhlbi.nih.gov

National Institute of Arthritis and Musculoskeletal and Skin Diseases (NIAMS)
1 AMS Cir.
Bethesda, MD 20892-3675
Toll-Free: 877-22-NIAMS
(877-226-4267)
Phone: 301-495-4484
TTY: 301-565-2966
Fax: 301-718-6366
Website: www.niams.nih.gov
Email: NIAMSinfo@mail.nih.gov

National Institute of Diabetes and Digestive and Kidney Diseases (NIDDK)
9000 Rockville Pike
Bethesda, MD 20892
Toll-Free: 800-860-8747
Toll-Free TTY: 866-569-1162
Website: www.niddk.nih.gov
Email: healthinfo@niddk.nih.gov

National Institute of Neurological Disorders and Stroke (NINDS)
P.O. Box 5801
Bethesda, MD 20824
Toll-Free: 800-352-9424
Phone: 301-496-5751
Website: www.ninds.nih.gov

National Institute on Aging (NIA)
31 Center Dr., MSC 2292
Bldg. 31, Rm. 5C27
Bethesda, MD 20892
Toll-Free: 800-222-2225
Phone: 301-496-1752
Toll-Free TTY: 800-222-4225
Website: www.nia.nih.gov
Email: niaic@nia.nih.gov

National Institutes of Health (NIH)
9000 Rockville Pike
Bethesda, MD 20892
Phone: 301-496-4000
TTY: 301-402-9612
Website: www.nih.gov

National Women's Health Information Center (NWHIC)
200 Independence Ave., S.W.
Rm. 712E
Washington, DC 20201
Toll-Free: 800-994-9662
Phone: 202-690-7650
Toll-Free TDD: 888-220-5446
Fax: 202-205-2631
Website: www.womenshealth.gov

U.S. Department of Health and Human Services (HHS)
200 Independence Ave., S.W.
Washington, DC 20201
Toll-Free: 877-696-6775
Website: www.hhs.gov

U.S. Food and Drug Administration (FDA)
10903 New Hampshire Ave.
Silver Spring, MD 20993
Toll-Free: 888-INFO-FDA
(888-463-6332)
Phone: 301-796-8240
Website: www.fda.gov

U.S. National Library of Medicine (NLM)
8600 Rockville Pike
Bethesda, MD 20894
Toll-Free: 888-FIND-NLM
(888-346-3656)
Phone: 301-594-5983
Website: www.nlm.nih.gov
Email: custserv@nlm.nih.gov

PRIVATE ORGANIZATIONS

Accreditation Association for Ambulatory Health Care (AAAHC)
3 Pkwy N., Ste. 201
Deerfield, IL 60015
Phone: 847-853-6060
Website: www.aaahc.org
Email: info@aaahc.org

Ambulatory Surgery Center Association (ASCA)
277 S. Washington St., Ste. 375
Alexandria, VA 22314
Phone: 703-836-8808
Website: www.ascassociation.org

American Academy of Cosmetic Surgery (AACS)
1932 S. Halsted St., Ste. 413
Chicago, IL 60608
Phone: 312-981-6760
Fax: 630-262-1520
Website: www.cosmeticsurgery.org
Email: info@cosmeticsurgery.org

American Academy of Dermatology (AAD)
P.O. Box 1968
Des Plaines, IL 60017
Toll-Free: 888-462-DERM (888-462-3376)
Phone: 847-240-1280
Fax: 847-240-1859
Website: www.aad.org

American Academy of Facial Plastic and Reconstructive Surgery (AAFPRS)
310 S. Henry St.
Alexandria, VA 22314
Phone: 703-299-9291
Fax: 703-299-8898
Website: www.aafprs.org
Email: info@aafprs.org

American Academy of Family Physicians (AAFP)
11400 Tomahawk Creek Pkwy
Leawood, KS 66211-2680
Toll-Free: 800-274-2237
Phone: 913-906-6000
Fax: 913-906-6075
Website: www.aafp.org

American Academy of Neurological and Orthopaedic Surgeons
1516 N. Lake Shore Dr.
Chicago, IL 60610
Phone: 312-787-1608
Fax: 312-787-9289
Website: aanos.org

American Academy of Ophthalmology (AAO)
655 Beach St.
San Francisco, CA 94109
Phone: 415-561-8500
Fax: 415-561-8533
Website: www.aao.org
Email: customer_service@aao.org

American Academy of Orthopaedic Surgeons (AAOS)
9400 W. Higgins Rd.
Rosemont, IL 60018
Phone: 847-823-7186
Fax: 847-823-8125
Website: www.aaos.org

American Academy of Otolaryngology—Head and Neck Surgery (AAO—HNS)
1650 Diagonal Rd.
Alexandria, VA 22314
Phone: 703-836-4444
Website: www.entnet.org

The American Association for the Surgery of Trauma
633 N. Saint Clair St.
Ste. 2600
Chicago, IL 60611
Toll-Free: 800-789-4006
Fax: 312-202-5064
Website: www.aast.org/Default.aspx
Email: aast@aast.org

American Association of Endodontists (AAE)
180 N. Stetson Ave., Ste. 1500
Chicago, IL 60601
Toll-Free: 800-872-3636
Phone: 312-266-7255
Fax: 312-266-9867
Toll-Free Fax: 866-451-9020
Website: www.aae.org
Email: info@aae.org

American Association of Hip and Knee Surgeons (AAHKS)
9400 W. Higgins Rd., Ste. 230
Rosemont, IL 60018-4976
Fax: 847-698-0704
Website: www.aahks.org

American Board of Cosmetic Surgery (ABCS)
8840 Calumet Ave., Ste. 205
Munster, IN 46321
Phone: 219-836-8585
Fax: 219-836-5525
Website: www.americanboardcosmeticsurgery.org

American Board of Plastic Surgery (ABPS)
1601 Market St.
Philadelphia, PA 19103-2204
Phone: 215-587-9322
Fax: 215-587-9622
Website: www.abplasticsurgery.org
Email: info@ABplasticsurgery.org

American Board of Surgery (ABS)
1617 John F. Kennedy Blvd., Ste. 860
Philadelphia, PA 19103
Phone: 215-568-4000
Fax: 215-563-5718
Website: www.absurgery.org

American Cancer Society (ACS)
270 Peachtree St., N.W., Ste. 1300
Atlanta, GA 30303
Toll-Free: 800-227-2345
Website: www.cancer.org

American College of Chest Physicians (CHEST)
2595 Patriot Blvd.
Glenview, IL 60026
Toll-Free: 800-343-2227
Phone: 224-521-9800
Fax: 224-521-9801
Website: www.chestnet.org

American College of Obstetricians and Gynecologists (ACOG)
409 12th St., S.W.
Washington, DC 20024-2188
Toll-Free: 800-673-8444
Phone: 202-638-5577
Website: www.acog.org
Email: resources@acog.org

American College of Radiology (ACR)
1892 Preston White Dr.
Reston, VA 20191
Toll-Free: 800-227-5463
Phone: 703-648-8900
Website: www.acr.org
Email: info@acr.org

American College of Surgeons (ACS)
633 N. Saint Clair St.
Chicago, IL 60611-3295
Toll-Free: 800-621-4111
Phone: 312-202-5000
Fax: 312-202-5001
Website: www.facs.org
Email: postmaster@facs.org

American Dental Association (ADA)
211 E. Chicago Ave.
Chicago, IL 60611-2678
Phone: 312-440-2500
Website: www.ada.org

American Heart Association (AHA)
7272 Greenville Ave.
Dallas, TX 75231
Toll-Free: 800-AHA-USA-1 (800-242-8721)
Website: www.heart.org

American Medical Association (AMA)
AMA Plaza 330 N., Wabash Ave.
Ste. 39300
Chicago, IL 60611-5885
Toll-Free: 800-262-3211
Website: www.ama-assn.org

American Optometric Association (AOA)
243 N. Lindbergh Blvd.
First Fl.
St. Louis, MO 63141-7881
Toll-Free: 800-365-2219
Phone: 314-991-4100
Website: www.aoa.org

American Pediatric Surgical Association (APSA)
1061 E. Main St., Ste. 300
East Dundee, IL 60118
Toll-Free: 309-PED-SURG (309-733-7874)
Phone: 847-686-2237
Website: apsapedsurg.org
Email: info@apsapedsurg.org

American Pregnancy Association
3007 Skyway Cir., N., Ste. 800
Irving, TX 75038
Toll-Free: 800-672-2296
Website: americanpregnancy.org
Email: info@americanpregnancy.org

American Psychological Association (APA)
750 First St., N.E.
Washington, DC 20002-4242
Toll-Free: 800-374-2721
Phone: 202-336-5500
TDD/TTY: 202-336-6123
Website: www.apa.org

American Rhinologic Society (ARS)
2820 N. Pinal Ave.
Casa Grande, AZ 85122
Phone: 973-545-2735
Website: www.american-rhinologic.org

American Society for Dermatologic Surgery (ASDS)
1933 N. Meacham Rd., Ste. 650
Schaumburg, IL 60173
Phone: 847-956-0900
Fax: 847-956-0999
Website: www.asds.net

American Society for Laser Medicine and Surgery (ASLMS)
100 N. 72nd Ave.
Wausau, WI 54401
Toll-Free: 877-258-6028
Phone: 715-845-9283
Website: www.aslms.org
Email: information@aslms.org

American Society for Metabolic and Bariatric Surgery (ASMBS)
14407 S.W. Second Pl., Ste. F-3
Newberry, FL 32669
Phone: 352-331-4900
Website: asmbs.org
Email: info@asmbs.org

American Society for Radiation Oncology (ASTRO)
251 18th St., S.
Eighth Fl.
Arlington, VA 22202
Phone: 703-502-1550
Fax: 703-502-7852
Website: www.astro.org

American Society for Reproductive Medicine (ASRM)
726 7th St. S.E.
Washington, DC 20003
Phone: 202-863-4985
Website: www.reproductivefacts.org

American Society for Surgery of the Hand (ASSH)
822 W. Washington Blvd.
Fl. 2
Chicago, IL 60607
Phone: 312-880-1900
Website: www.assh.org
Email: info@assh.org

American Society of Anesthesiologists (ASA)
1061 American Ln.
Schaumburg, IL 60173-4973
Phone: 847-825-5586
Fax: 847-825-1692
Website: www.asahq.org
Email: info@asahq.org

American Society of Colon and Rectal Surgeons (ASCRS)
2515 Waukegan Rd., Ste. 210
Bannockburn, IL 60015
Phone: 847-607-6410
Website: fascrs.org
Email: ascrs@fascrs.org

American Society of Ophthalmic Plastic and Reconstructive Surgery (ASOPRS)
1041 Grand Ave., Ste. 132
St Paul, MN 55105
Phone: 612-601-3168
Website: www.asoprs.org
Email: info@asoprs.org

American Society of PeriAnesthesia Nurses (ASPAN)
90 Frontage Rd.
Cherry Hill, NJ 08034-1424
Toll-Free: 877-737-9696
Fax: 856-616-9601
Website: www.aspan.org
Email: aspan@aspan.org

American Society of Plastic Surgeons (ASPS)
444 E. Algonquin Rd.
Arlington Heights, IL 60005
Phone: 847-228-9900
Website: www.plasticsurgery.org
Email: memserv@plasticsurgery.org

American Society of Transplantation (AST)
1000 Atrium Way
Mt. Laurel, NJ 08054
Phone: 856-439-9986
Fax: 856-581-9604
Website: www.myast.org

American Thoracic Society (ATS)
25 Bdwy.
New York, NY 10004
Phone: 212-315-8600
Fax: 212-315-6498
Website: www.thoracic.org
Email: atsinfo@thoracic.org

American Thyroid Association (ATA)
2000 Duke St., Ste. 300
Alexandria, VA 22314
Website: www.thyroid.org

Amputee Coalition of America (ACA)
601 Pennsylvania Ave.
N.W., Ste. 420
South Bldg.
Washington, DC 20004
Toll-Free: 888-267-5669
Website: www.amputee-coalition.org

Arthritis Foundation® (AF)
1355 Peachtree St., N.E., Ste. 600
Atlanta, GA 30309
Toll-Free: 800-283-7800
Website: www.arthritis.org

Association for Academic Surgery (AAS)
11300 W. Olympic Blvd., Ste. 600
Los Angeles, CA 90064
Phone: 310-437-1606
Fax: 310-437-0585
Website: www.aasurg.org
Email: admin@aasurg.org

Association of American Physicians and Surgeons (AAPS)
1601 N. Tucson Blvd., Ste. 9
Tucson, AZ 85716
Toll-Free: 800-635-1196
Fax: 520-325-4230
Website: aapsonline.org
Email: aaps@aapsonline.org

Eastern Association for the Surgery of Trauma
633 N. Saint Clair St., Ste. 2400
Chicago, IL 60611-3295
Phone: 312-202-5508
Fax: 312-202-5064
Website: www.east.org
Email: managementoffice@east.org

The Joint Commission
One Renaissance Blvd.
Oakbrook Terrace, IL 60181
Phone: 630-792-5800
Website: www.jointcommission.org

Mayo Foundation for Medical Education and Research (MFMER)
200 First St., S.W.
Rochester, MN 55905
Phone: 507-284-2511
Fax: 507-538-7802
Website: www.mayoclinic.org

National Hospice and Palliative Care Organization (NHPCO)
1731 King St.
Alexandria, VA 22314
Toll-Free: 800-658-8898
Phone: 703-837-1500
Fax: 703-837-1233
Website: www.nhpco.org

Planned Parenthood Federation of America (PPFA)
114 University Ave.
Rochester, NY 14605
Phone: 585-546-2595
Website: www.plannedparenthood.org

The Plastic Surgery Foundation (PSF)
444 E. Algonquin Rd.
Arlington Heights, IL 60005-4664
Toll-Free: 800-766-4955
Phone: 847-228-9900
Website: www.thepsf.org

Society of Critical Care Medicine (SCCM)
500 Midway Dr.
Mount Prospect, IL 60056
Phone: 847-827-6888
Fax: 847-439-7226
Website: www.sccm.org
Email: support@sccm.org

Society of Interventional Radiology (SIR)
3975 Fair Ridge Dr., Ste. 400 N.
Fairfax, VA 22033
Phone: 703-691-1805
Fax: 703-691-1855
Website: www.sirweb.org

Society of Nuclear Medicine and Molecular Imaging (SNMMI)
1850 Samuel Morse Dr.
Reston, VA 20190
Phone: 703-708-9000
Fax: 703-708-9015
Website: www.snmmi.org

Society of Thoracic Surgeons (STS)
633 N. Saint Clair St., Ste. 2100
Chicago, IL 60611
Phone: 312-202-5800
Fax: 312-202-5801
Website: www.sts.org

Texas Heart Institute (THI)
6770 Bertner Ave.
Houston, TX 77030
Phone: 832-355-3792
Website: www.texasheart.org

United Network for Organ Sharing (UNOS)
700 N. Fourth St.
Richmond, VA 23219
Toll-Free: 800-292-9548
Phone: 804-782-4800
Fax: 804-782-4817
Website: www.unos.org
Email: patientservices@unos.org

United Ostomy Associations of America, Inc. (UOAA)
P.O. Box 2293
Biddeford, ME 04005-2293
Toll-Free: 800-826-0826
Website: www.ostomy.org
Email: info@ostomy.org

INDEX

INDEX

Page numbers followed by "n" refer to citation information; by "t" indicate tables; and by "f" indicate figures.

A

Index

B

C

Index

D

H

M

O

P

Q

R

V

W